The Orthopedic Educator

Paul J. Dougherty
Barbara L. Joyce
Editors

The Orthopedic Educator

A Pocket Guide

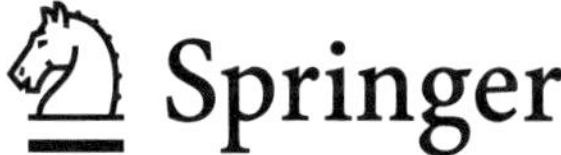 Springer

Editors
Paul J. Dougherty
College of
  Medicine-Jacksonville
Department of Orthopaedic
  Surgery, University of Florida
Jacksonville, FL
USA

Barbara L. Joyce
William Beaumont School of
  Medicine
Oakland University
Rochester, MI
USA

ISBN 978-3-319-62943-8   ISBN 978-3-319-62944-5   (eBook)
DOI 10.1007/978-3-319-62944-5

Library of Congress Control Number: 2017956810

This Springer imprint is published by Springer Nature
The registered company is Springer International Publishing AG
The registered company address is: Gewerbestrasse 11, 6330 Cham, Switzerland

Preface

There are hundreds of books about orthopaedic surgery. The vast majority deal with evaluation and treatment of specific orthopaedic problems, especially steps in surgical techniques. This book is different; it is about providing education to orthopaedic surgeons. Other books exist about medical education, they are more focused on medical students or the medical specialties. While there are a number of common aspects to teaching in all specialties, surgical specialties differ in that competence is developed in the care of surgical patients and performing surgical procedures.

Surgical education, and in this case orthopaedic surgery, differs from nonsurgical specialties in that competence also means being able to perform surgery consistently in a competent manner. Furthermore, the increased burden of reporting, documentation, and time constraints have made being an orthopaedic educator more complex. Twenty years ago, little preparation was needed to become a program director. Today it requires a solid understanding of educational principals, ACGME requirements, and leadership.

The purpose of this book is to provide a single source, in a concise manner, a resource for those who provide education to medical students, residents, and faculty development for the department educators of an orthopaedic department. The chapters cover the evolution of orthopaedic surgery residency, how orthopaedic surgery is taught in other countries, curriculum development, residency organization, feedback for residents, resident assessment, remediation, teaching surgical skills, faculty development, and medical student education. We hope this volume provides a solid foundation for those who provide graduate medical education for residency programs, including educators, faculty, and program directors and aspiring residents.

Jacksonville, FL   Paul J. Dougherty, MD
Rochester, MI   Barbara L. Joyce, PhD

Editors' Biography

Paul J. Dougherty, MD is Professor and Chairman of the Department of Orthopaedic Surgery at the University of Florida College of Medicine-Jacksonville, as well as the residency Program Director. He has been a residency program director for the past 19 years, spanning military, university, and managed care environments. As part of this, he has graduated over eighty orthopaedic surgeons to practice. Dr. Dougherty is a retired US Army Colonel, who deployed to Somalia and Afghanistan during his career. He has been the editor for the American Academy of Orthopaedic Surgeons monograph entitled *Gunshot Wounds*, as well as being on the editorial board for the *NATO Emergency War Surgery Handbook, 4th US edition*, which describes the initial care of battlefield injuries.

Dr. Dougherty received his MD from Uniformed Services School of Medicine, located in Bethesda, Maryland. He did his surgical internship at William Beaumont Army Medical Center in El Paso, Texas. His orthopaedic residency was conducted at Letterman Army Medical Center in San Francisco, followed by the Oakland Naval Hospital after Letterman closed due to downsizing of the US military. Dr. Dougherty subsequently completed an Orthopaedic Trauma Fellowship at the University of Louisville, in Louisville, Kentucky.

Currently, Dr. Dougherty has an education column which is published quarterly in *Clinical Orthopaedics and Related Research*. He has over 50 published peer-reviewed publications, in the areas of orthopaedic trauma, education, amputee care, and wound ballistics.

He is a Member-at-Large for the Council of Orthopaedic Residency Directors (CORD) and is also an oral examiner for the American Board of Orthopaedic Surgery Part 2 Certifying Examinations.

Barbara L. Joyce, PhD is the Director of Curriculum Evaluation and Associate Professor of Biomedical Science at Oakland University William Beaumont School of Medicine. She is responsible for the evaluation of the medical school curriculum, promoting faculty excellence and innovation in curricular development, and scholarly activity.

Dr. Joyce was the Director of Instructional Design at Henry Ford Health System and Clinical Associate Professor in the Department of Family Medicine at Wayne State University. She was responsible for designing, implementing, and evaluating curricula, assessment tools, and program improvement processes for 45 ACGME accredited residency and fellowship training programs. She was also responsible for designing educational curricula, assessment tools, and program improvement process for the Henry Ford Health System Center for Simulation Education and Research. Prior to this position, she was Senior Project Manager at the ACGME where she worked on the Outcome Project and provided faculty development on the ACGME competencies. Her additional past experiences have been as Associate Director of Behavioral Science at Genesys Regional Medical Center where she was responsible for Family Medicine resident training and training of Health Psychology postdoctoral fellows, and Director of Behavioral Science at Sinai Hospital in Detroit. She has spoken nationally and internationally on competency-based education in graduate medical education. Dr. Joyce is a clinical psychologist.

Contents

Contributors

Jaimo Ahn, MD, PhD The Corporal Michael J. Crescenz VA Medical Center and The University of Pennsylvania Perelman School of Medicine, Philadelphia, PA, USA

Joseph Bernstein, MD The Corporal Michael J. Crescenz VA Medical Center and The University of Pennsylvania Perelman School of Medicine, Philadelphia, PA, USA

Marlene A. DeMaio, MD Department of Orthopaedic Surgery, Perelman School of Medicine, University of Pennsylvania, Philadelphia, PA, USA

Paul J. Dougherty, MD Department of Orthopaedic Surgery, University of Florida College of Medicine — Jacksonville, Jacksonville, FL, USA

Paul G. Echols, MD Department of Orthopaedics and Rehabilitation, The University of New Mexico Health Sciences Center, Albuquerque, NM, USA

S. Elizabeth Ames, MD Department of Orthopaedics and Rehabilitation, The Robert Larner, MD College of Medicine, University of Vermont, Burlington, VT, USA

Barbara L. Joyce, PhD Oakland University William Beaumont School of Medicine, Rochester, MI, USA

Matthew D. Karam, MD The Department of Orthopedics and Rehabilitation, The University of Iowa Hospitals and Clinics, Iowa City, IA, USA

J. Lawrence Marsh, MD The Department of Orthopedics and Rehabilitation, The University of Iowa Hospitals and Clinics, Iowa City, IA, USA

Kathleen McHale, MD, MSEd George Washington University, Uniformed Services University for the Health Sciences, Alexandria, VA, USA

Deana M. Mercer, MD Department of Orthopaedics and Rehabilitation, The University of New Mexico Health Sciences Center, Albuquerque, NM, USA

Martin J. Morrison III, MD Loma Linda University Medical Center, Loma Linda, CA, USA

Nathaniel Nelms, MD Department of Orthopaedics and Rehabilitation, The Robert Larner, MD College of Medicine, University of Vermont, Burlington, VT, USA

Donna Phillips, MD Orthopaedic Surgery and Pediatrics, Chief Pediatric Orthopedic Surgery Bellevue Hospital, Bellevue Hospital, New York, NY, USA

Craig S. Roberts, MD, MBA Department of Orthopaedic Surgery Academic Office, University of Louisville School of Medicine, Louisville, KY, USA

Vani Sabesan, MD Department of Orthopaedic Surgery, Beaumont Health System/Wayne State University, Dearborn, MI, USA

Robert C. Schenck Jr., MD Department of Orthopaedics and Rehabilitation, The University of New Mexico Health Sciences Center, Albuquerque, NM, USA

Hasan M. Syed, MD Loma Linda University Medical Center, Loma Linda, CA, USA

A.E. Van Heest, MD Department of Orthopaedic Surgery, University of Minnesota, Minneapolis, MN, USA

Daniel C. Wascher, MD Department of Orthopaedics and Rehabilitation, The University of New Mexico Health Sciences Center, Albuquerque, NM, USA

James Whaley, MD Department of Orthopaedic Surgery, Wayne State University, Cleveland Clinic, Weston, FL, USA

M. Daniel Wongworawat, MD Loma Linda University Medical Center, Loma Linda, CA, USA

Chapter 1
History of Orthopaedic Surgery Residency in the United States

Paul J. Dougherty

Introduction

Beginning with a nascent few programs a hundred years ago, to over 155 separate residency programs today, there has been an evolution of residency program structure, content, and pedagogy that has served to educate new doctors into trained specialists. The purpose of this chapter is to review the changes and content for orthopaedic surgery and to document the changes in the structure and practice of orthopaedic education with a particular focus on how orthopaedic surgery has been taught within the residency program. What were the structural changes that took place over time? With advances in the field, how did the content change over time? What methods were used to provide education of residents? By viewing orthopaedic surgery residency programs in this longitudinal fashion, it potentially provides us a road map in providing future direction to residency programs.

P.J. Dougherty, MD
Department of Orthopaedic Surgery, University of Florida
College of Medicine—Jacksonville, 655 W 8th Street,
2nd Floor ACC, Jacksonville, FL 32209, USA
e-mail: paul.dougherty@jax.ufl.edu

© Springer International Publishing AG 2018
P.J. Dougherty, B.L. Joyce (eds.), *The Orthopedic Educator*,
DOI 10.1007/978-3-319-62944-5_1

Origins of Residency

The idea of a formal residency has its origins with the formation of formal surgical residencies at Johns Hopkins at the turn of the last century. Combined with advancements in this field of orthopaedic surgery, the recognition of an increasingly sophisticated specialty led to the development of an orthopaedic residency by William Baer M.D. along the lines of the one created by William Halstead M.D. Baer was a graduate of the Halstead residency, and was encouraged by Halstead to develop this new field of orthopaedic surgery. Baer set up an orthopaedic outpatient clinic in 1900 at Johns Hopkins and established a residency program, with its first graduate in 1915. There was one graduate per year until Baer's death in 1931 [1]. Osgood at Massachusetts General Hospital followed in a similar vein in the early 1920s, but established a residency that was of a prescribed length: 1-year children's, 1-year adult, and 6 months' basic science education [2].

Slow development of all specialty education occurred during the 1920s and 1930s. There were three commonly accepted ways of obtaining specialty training. First, doctors who had already been in practice could attend a "short course" of orthopaedic surgery, receiving didactics, and perhaps perform surgical procedures on an animal model. Second, there was the preceptorship model in which a doctor practiced with someone in the specialty, learning about the specialty over time. Third, there was the development of residency programs which gradually increased over time and ultimately displaced the other two methods as a means for education. Residencies gradually became more common as a superior method of education (as opposed to preceptorship or short courses) from 1920 to 1945 as a means of standardizing education for specialties. In conjunction with the development of education was board certification of all specialties. The American Board of Orthopaedic Surgery (ABOS) was incorporated in 1934, around the same time as the fields of general surgery, internal medicine, and ophthalmology. The ABOS initially had the role of accreditation and approval of residency programs.

The 1936 "Rules and Procedures" of the American Board of Orthopaedic Surgery stipulated new conditions, to go in effect after 1938, for qualification of Board Certification to be: " … three years of concentrated instruction in orthopaedic surgery approved by and acceptable to the board." and " … have had two years of further clinical experience in the actual practice of orthopaedic surgery." and "… must have knowledge of the basic medical sciences related to orthopaedic surgery [3].

By 1943 the requirements had been further refined to " … have served for an approved period … an internship in a general hospital approved by the Board" and " … should have served as resident for three years in an orthopaedic surgery or fellowship in a hospital or medical school approved by this Board." Additionally, the curriculum should include " … instruction in the related basic sciences, orthopaedic surgery, of adults and children and the treatment of fractures" [4]. By 1946, the American Board of Orthopaedic Surgery had set educational criteria for residency programs.

World War II caused the mobilization of an unprecedented number of doctors. For example, the US Army went from about 1200 at the time of Pearl Harbor and peaking at about 47,000 by the end of the war. Returning doctors from overseas, as well as new medical school graduates, were interested in specialty training, which necessitated the need for approved "training services" by both the ABOS and AMA. By May 1949, there were 257 approved services listed for a total of 787 positions. Positions at hospitals were divided into adult, children, fracture, and basic sciences [5].

What then was the scope or content of orthopaedic surgery at this time? Willis Campbell M.D. was chairman of the Campbell clinic in the 1930s and wrote a comprehensive textbook entitled "Operative Orthopaedics" which was published in 1939. This textbook is updated with new editions every seven or so years, and is now in its 13th Edition. With some limitations, it has been a consistent barometer for procedures conducted by practicing orthopaedic surgeons, and a guidebook for those in training. From the first edition of 1200 pages, the text has grown to now four volumes and 4766 pages [6, 7].

The first edition was published at the beginning of World War II for Europe (1939) but 2 years before US involvement in the war. Described in this edition were 635 surgical procedures (this number does not include the chapters on "surgical approaches"). Included in the volume were chapters about the treatment of polio and acute and chronic bone infection. Large chapters were devoted to the treatment of fracture malunions or nonunions.

The second edition came out in 1949 and had grown to two volumes and approximately 1700 pages in length. Included in the introduction was the encouragement of the editors to use the book as a guide for residency training. There were approximately 740 procedures listed, including the new "mold arthroplasty" of the hip to treat hip arthritis. For the treatment of fractures, more extensive description of plates and screws was made, along with a description of the new intramedullary nailing of diaphyseal fractures [8].

It is evident that a great deal of thought went into the content of education, including the clinical problems to be treated, the requisite basic sciences involved, and rehabilitation. In establishing the early residencies, educators also advocated progressive responsibility [5]. Dana Street, M.D. wrote about a program he established for the Veterans Administration in 1949, stating that in a resident's final 6 months "he is in complete charge of the ward, and does most of the surgery on patients …." Street explained after rotating as a junior resident, and assisting on cases, that the senior resident "is supervised for the first case by faculty, and depending on the residents' aptitude, may be allowed to operate without direct supervision." More complicated cases were performed with faculty [9].

William Green M.D., at Boston Children's Hospital, wrote that an ideal rotation would have enough clinical material in order to train residents in all facets of patient care. Furthermore, he recognized that hands-on or active learning needed to take place and stated: "The men in training should do the work; observation is of limited value." Progressive, structured independence for resident education was necessary to ensure that someone was competent at the end of their training. Green recommended resident autonomy coupled with good supervision. "The teaching of surgery must be well supervised. Training should evolve through assisting and performing operative procedures assisted by a competent teacher, with progression to more independence as a senior resident. A man cannot learn surgery unless he does it" [10, p. 890].

Accreditation

The Residency Review Committee (RRC) for orthopaedic surgery was formed in 1953 as a committee with representation from the ABOS and the orthopaedic section of the AMA. The RRC's purpose was to accredit residency programs in the United States. The Liaison Committee on Graduate Medical Education provided oversight to all medical specialty RRCs beginning in 1972. The AAOS had representation on the RRC beginning in 1973. These three components, ABOS, AAOS, and AMA, have representation on the current RRC, which has been under the Accreditation Council on Graduate Medical Education (ACGME) since 1981.

1950s and 1960s

Orthopaedic practice continued to slowly advance in the 1950s and 1960s. Requirements of a residency program consisted of a preliminary year (or 2) and 3 years of orthopaedic education.

The 1956 edition of *Campbell's Operative Orthopaedics* had grown to 2124 p. in two volumes, expanding to descriptions of nearly 850 procedures. Polio and skeletal tuberculosis were still prevalent, and surgeries to care for them were still included. The new editors, however, emphasized indications and contraindications for procedures in caring for patients. The chapters on fracture malunions and nonunions, as well as nerve injuries and amputations, were expanded based on experience and improvements in caring for those types of patients during and after the Second World War [11].

Orthopaedic surgery was developing as a surgical specialty in its own right, and by the early 1960s there were concerns about the loss of part of the specialty to other disciplines. Orthopaedic surgery had traditionally been responsible for nonoperative care as well, and there was concern about the loss of the rehabilitation aspect of the specialty to the developing field of rehabilitation. Additionally, there was a tradition in some institutions for general surgery to also care for patients with acute fractures, along with orthopaedic surgery. This loss of parts of the specialty to other disciplines was noted with concern by orthopaedic leaders, who felt that continuing to define orthopaedic surgery as a single broad specialty was important. Such "turf wars" continue today, with spine care being part of both orthopaedic and neurosurgery, for example. Fracture care is now strictly the domain of orthopaedic surgery, whereas rehabilitation has developed into its own specialty of Physical Medicine and Rehabilitation (12).

J. Vernon Luck, who was President of the American Academy of Orthopaedic Surgeons, proposed in 1961 that after internship, an orthopaedic residency should consist of 2 1/2 years of adult and child orthopaedic surgery, orthopaedic trauma, hand surgery, rehabilitation, and basic science. For someone going into a teaching program, he recommended another 1–2 years in one of the areas so the resident could obtain proficiency in that area. For someone who was not going into academics, the last year would be balanced senior rotations of the above-named areas. A second track would consist of continued rotations and general orthopaedic surgery for the resident who was going into a general orthopaedic surgery practice [12]. Robinson, Chairman of the Orthopaedic program at Johns Hopkins, felt that offering a research year within the orthopaedic residency would be a way to enhance the academic credentials of a resident. He did not feel that this program should be offered to all residents, but more to those who want to do academic medicine [13].

The 1963 edition of *Campbell's Operative Orthopaedics* was 1778 pages in two volumes. There were 925 separate procedures described. Included in this edition was a new comprehensive chapter on hand surgery, as well as a new editor, AH Crenshaw [14].

Residency programs were evolving as to resident experience as well, and while no two programs were exactly alike, some common experiences emerged. First, the total complement of residents ranged from two to four per year group in most programs, with programs greater than four per year group being rare. The number of faculty was also fewer, with some programs having 2–4 full-time faculty members at the home institution. Resident rotations would often encompass working at a county or university hospital for the majority of the residency, but they also rotated with select surgeons in private practice to learn about other techniques. Furthermore, a required part of the residency was to be exclusively pediatric orthopaedic surgery, often rotating at a pediatric hospital. Within the main institution, there were often resident-run clinics which were exclusively supported by residents who would make all decisions about patient care. Residents saw patients with fractures or infections in these clinics. While faculty were available for consultation, the autonomy provided by these rotations allowed for residents to learn how to care for patients independently.

In 1963 the American Academy of Orthopaedic Surgeons offered residents the first in-service examination. This exam was for residents, provided as a means to practice a written exam in the format of the ABOS written certification exams. It was to provide feedback to the resident, as well as the program, about how well the program was providing overall education about orthopaedic knowledge. The Orthopaedic In-Training Exam or "OITE" has been given continuously since 1963, and most program directors find this a useful measure about their resident's performance relative to the rest of the programs in the country [15]. Additionally, the exam has been shown to correlate to the ABOS Part 1 certifying examination [16].

Orthopaedic surgery became better defined during the 1960s, and as a result residents would have rotations on a general orthopaedic service, possibly hand, and children's services. Formal musculoskeletal pathology courses were also developing as a means to provide resident education (and those reviewing for their ABOS exams) about musculoskeletal oncology, bone infections, and noninfectious diseases (like Rickets).

There were some outstanding educators. James E Johnson, M.D., provided generations of orthopaedic surgery residents in the San Francisco Bay Area a yearly musculoskeletal review course in the evenings over several weeks prior to the OITE exams. (There were two military programs, a program at St. Mary's Hospital and the University of California at San Francisco.) He was known for a teaching style in which a resident was given a pointer (in the latter years, this was a laser pointer) shown a 35 mm slide of an X-ray of a patient, and asked successively more detailed questions, until the differential diagnosis had been obtained along with a treatment plan determined. For the next patient example, the pointer would get passed along. Appropriately, he was awarded the "best teacher" award for several years by the University of California San Francisco residents. He also provided an intense review for those in June for those preparing for their ABOS exams.

Philip D. Wilson M.D., President of the American Academy of Orthopaedic Surgeons, editorialized in 1973 about the deficiencies in the education and certification process [17]. He noted: "the first is the failure of our residency programs to weed out those relatively few individuals with problems of attitude or with deficiency of psychomotor skills before they reach the board exam level. The second is the inability, thus far, to develop examination methods to measure reliably these two important parameters of an orthopedic surgeon's competence [17, p. 861]."

Educators felt in the late 1970s that orthopaedic surgery was becoming a larger specialty, requiring more education [20]. In 1978, an extra year was added by the American Board of Orthopaedic Surgeons to the residency program, allowing for 4 years of residency following internship. The internship itself was to provide a broad base of education. This was in response to a perceived increase in the scope of the specialty.

1980s

By 1980, new technologies and procedures had evolved for orthopaedic surgery. Orthopaedic surgeons were beginning to perform arthroscopy of the knee, and total knee and total hip arthroplasties were becoming more common. Fracture care also became more sophisticated during the 1980s. Intramedullary nailing of the tibia, femur, and humerus became more common, for example. Open reduction, internal fixation became a more reliable procedure, involving periarticular fractures, including those of the acetabulum.

For the 1980 edition, *Campbell's Operative Orthopaedics* had grown to 2435 pages in two volumes, with a new editor, AE Edmondson, working with the previous editor AW Crenshaw [18]. Included was an expanded chapter of hip and knee arthroplasty and a larger chapter on hand surgery, as well as an expanded section on fracture care [17].

William Enneking M.D., an orthopaedic surgeon who specialized in musculoskeletal oncology at the University of Florida, also known as an outstanding educator of medical students, residents, fellows, and practicing orthopaedic surgeons, noted changes occurring in the practice of orthopaedic surgery in the early 1980s which were concerning. As a long-time orthopaedic oral examiner for the ABOS, he noted a change which gradually occurred in the quality of those sitting for the examinations. While most were competent, there was a palpable group that was clearly not prepared for practice. He attributed this decline to a number of factors, including resident selection and assessment of residents during their education [19].

An orthopaedic resident's experience in the 1980s emphasized more surgery than in previous generations, because of the advances seen in the operative management of a number of conditions. While supervision was increased, there still were rotations for many programs which were very resident dependent. One example is of the Wayne County Hospital, a county hospital which served the area near Detroit, Michigan. One former resident describes being on every other night call, and on the nights off not leaving the hospital until 9 p.m. She notes that this rotation was "a rite of passage" for the residents, and that reputations were made based on the ability to rotate successfully at the county hospital. Patients were managed by residents in the clinic, with faculty available for consultation. Furthermore, decisions to operate were made by residents, with faculty consultation if needed.

1990s

The 8th edition of *Campbell's Operative Orthopaedics* (A.H. Crenshaw, Ed) was published in 1992 with five volumes and 3790 p., following relatively quickly the 1987 edition [21]. There were several developments in the new edition, with newer techniques (for example the inclusion of pedicle screws for spine surgery, expanded foot and ankle and fracture care). This edition is important, because of the procedures described within the text. Procedures that are part of general orthopaedic education have not perceptibly changed since this edition. While some subspecialty items have changed, common procedures to treat hip and knee arthritis, rotator cuff tear, hip fracture stabilization, and anterior cruciate ligament disruption are the same today.

The rise of subspecialization (see below) took place beginning in the 1980s and continues today. This led to an increased proportion of orthopaedic surgeons taking fellowships for the purpose of having a subset of specialized skills, which also influenced teaching faculty in residency programs. As teaching faculty became more specialized, there was a gradual shift from a general orthopaedic practice towards subspecialty rotations, thus differentiating the character in some programs away from what was seen in an average orthopaedic practice at that time.

As teaching faculty at residency programs increased, some programs expanded their resident complement, with large programs having 8–12 residents per year group (40–60 total residents in a program). These larger programs, though having more faculty, did not allow for the close relationships to develop previously as seen with smaller programs. Larger programs also tended to have shorter rotations, therefore allowing less time with the faculty member that had previously been seen.

Residency programs gradually began to have more subspecialization as well. For example, previous residency programs would have a general adult service or services, whose goal was to treat a wide variety of clinical problems on a single team. While exceptions existed, a gradual restructuring of residency programs to more subspecialty-based rotations (spine, trauma, adult reconstruction, sports, and foot and ankle) led to a loss of what a residency graduate would experience within a general orthopaedic practice. Additionally, nonoperative treatment or management was gradually de-emphasized in residency programs, as part of the increased operative treatment of orthopaedic problems as well as a de-emphasis on nonoperative care in practices.

2000 Onward

Public outcry about the hours worked by residents, publicized by high-profile cases such as the Libby Zion case in New York City, had been a focus since the early 1980s. With the publication of the Institute of Medicines report *To Err is Human* in 1999, in which the authors concluded that there were potentially 48–98,000 deaths due to preventable errors in US hospitals, increased awareness in quality improvement and patient safety became part of the training environment [22].

As part of this, there was increasing public pressure to reduce duty hours as an effort to improve patient safety. As a result, duty-hour restrictions (<80 total hours/week, no more than 24 h on duty at a time, no more than 1/3 call, >10-h break between work days, and an average of 1:7 days off over 4 weeks) were implemented in 2003 [23]. At this point in time, there does not seem to be discernable difference between procedures done, OITE exam results, or patient safety [24]. So, while quality of life may have been improved, it does not appear that educational quality or patient care by residents has perceptibly changed with the duty-hour changes. Interestingly, national data does suggest that the average number of hours worked by orthopaedic residents does not approach 80 h per week. Other specialties, such as neurosurgery and general surgery, have more problems meeting these requirements. More recent changes, such as limiting PGY1s to no more than 16 h per day with no 24-h call, have been met with more resistance. As a result of the study, this last restriction was lifted at the beginning of this academic year (2016).

The six general competencies (patient care, communication and interpersonal skills, practice-based learning and improvement, systems-based practice, medical knowledge, and professionalism) were implemented by the ACGME in 2003 as a means to teach and assess residents in six domains of competence, regardless of the specialty. The Outcome Project was initiated as a means to both guide teaching and provide a means of assessment needed by every physician in any specialty. The major weakness was that the ACGME or RRCs did not provide educational content or assessment tools for any of the specialties. As a result, individual programs were left to develop both content and assessment tools on their own. This led to a great deal of dissatisfaction, and little useful data on how proficient graduates were in these six domains upon graduation [25].

In an effort to overcome these deficiencies, the Next Accreditation System (NAS) was developed to help define the progression of skills a resident should accomplish in order to complete a program in any specialty. Because differing specialties had their own content or topics for patient care and medical knowledge, each specialty RRC was tasked to develop a progression of standards, called milestones, for certain topics within the specialty. For patient care and medical knowledge, the specialties developed topics and expectations for performance at various levels of education, beginning from a novice to a resident who is ready to graduate. A consensus panel, having members of all orthopaedic subspecialties, chose 16 topics which were thought to represent a cross section of orthopaedic surgery. Beginning in the 2013–2014 academic year with Phase 1 programs (orthopaedic surgery was one), residents were to be assessed in the six general competencies with defined general expectations at differing levels of training in the program. Milestone evaluations for every resident are reported every 6 months for what rotations have been done over the previous 6 months. Within the individual program, the milestone evaluations were made by a new committee, the Clinical Competency Committee, which consists of faculty only who utilize all resident evaluations (from faculty, patients, nursing, OITE, procedure logs, etc.) to determine what progress a resident has made during the previous 6 months [25].

Operative procedure data was recorded and reported beginning in 2004, in which the reported procedures were tabulated for the program and compared nationally. Using data from the graduates, the RRC looks at reported overall procedure logs to determine whether the scope and breadth of procedures are adequate, when compared to programs in the rest of the country. Beginning in 2012, case volume minimums were also recorded in 15 categories, thought to represent common procedures in general orthopaedic surgery (for example, hip and knee arthroplasty, carpal tunnel release, and hip fractures).

Categorical Orthopaedic Internship

At this same time, the orthopaedic categorical internship was implemented in 2013, which increased the number of months for orthopaedic surgery rotations from 3 to 6 months in the

PGY1 year. By having an increased number of orthopaedic surgery rotations, an earlier exposure to orthopaedic surgery was thought to be beneficial, given the increased complexity of residency. By decreasing the rotations on general surgery specialties to allow for more orthopaedic rotations may have had unintended consequences, however. General surgery had much greater difficulty adjusting to the duty-hour requirements, and lessening the pool of available interns to work on those services intensified the crisis for general surgery interns and duty hours. Additionally, the specialization of the internship, while better for orthopaedic exposure, did not allow for those who did not match into orthopaedics but took another internship, to match into a PGY2 slot if there was an opening in an orthopaedic program [26].

Also beginning in the 2013–2014 academic year, ABOS initiated a program of intern surgical skills composed of 17 modules for introduction to key surgical skills. Topics included internal and external fixation, adult reconstruction, suturing and knot tying, team training and patient safety, fluoroscopic imaging, and operating room setup. All residency programs were to conduct this education, using the modules provided by the ABOS, to provide a comprehensive foundation for earlier orthopaedic surgical education [26].

Clinical Learning Environment

The Next Accreditation System also initiated Clinical Learning Environment Review (CLER) as part of a broader initiative to focus on continued improvements in the educational learning environment. Institutions were evaluated on how well they provided support in a clinical learning environment. While this included duty-hour compliance at the institution, they provided oversight for patient safety and quality improvement, in particular looking at transitions to care, professionalism, and supervision. While this oversight was managed by the institution's Graduate Medical Education office, orthopaedic surgery residents are expected to participate in quality improvement projects and have designated curriculum focused on quality improvement and patient safety [27].

The Rise of Fellowships

As the field of orthopaedic surgery has become more complex, there has been an increase in subspecialization. Hand surgery was the first fellowship that evolved after World War II, as a field to *combine* the expertise of plastic surgery, neurosurgery, and orthopaedic surgery. Sterling Bunnell, M.D., was asked by the US Army Surgeon General, Norman T. Kirk, M.D., to help set up specialty centers for hand surgery at Army Hospitals throughout the country [28]. Dr. Bunnell closed his practice in San Francisco and toured the Army hospitals which were considered hand referral centers, providing education for surgical management and rehabilitation of hand problems. The American Society for Surgery of the Hand held its first annual meeting in 1946, and its members were composed of doctors who ran the first hand centers for the Army. Subsequently, hand surgery fellowships were open to those in plastics, orthopaedic, and general surgery. While hand surgery was the first subspecialty, orthopaedic surgery remained largely the realm of the core specialty.

Subspecialization in orthopaedic surgery began in the 1970s with the advent of the American Society of Sports Medicine (1972), followed by a Musculoskeletal Tumor Society (1977). The 1980s saw initial meetings for the Pediatric Orthopaedic Society of North America (1983), the North American Spine Society (1985), and the Orthopaedic Trauma Association (1987). The Association of Hip and Knee Surgeons was formed in 1991.

The rise in fellowships led to concern about how educating fellows would influence the core residency program. Educators were divided on the effects of fellows on resident education, some describing a positive teaching effect for the residency program, whereas others felt that resident participation in cases is lessened [29–32]. Because of this, the

ACGME began accreditation for fellowships (hand, pediatric orthopaedics, trauma, sports, musculoskeletal tumor, and adult reconstruction) in the 1980s [30]. Spine and foot and ankle accreditation was offered in the early 1990s.

In mid-1995, approximately 62% of those taking the American Board of Orthopaedic Surgeons Part II Certifying Examinations reported having fellowships of at least a year in length [30]. In 2013, 90% of those taking the Part II exam had taken a fellowship [33]. Reasons for taking a fellowship are multifactorial. Some residents apply because they feel that it enhances their "marketability" to find a job after training. Others apply to enhance their skill set in a subspecialized field, hoping to practice in that field upon graduation. Another reason offered is that an individual residency program may be lacking in certain educational opportunities for a resident and therefore must be made up postgraduation. Urbaniak cited the growth of faculty at academic medical centers, with his own Duke program increasing 400% in the previous 25 years, yet with a decrease of 30% in residents [32]. Certain aspects of a fellowship appeal to subspecialized faculty. The fellow is more capable to handle more aspects of patient care, therefore allowing them to act as extenders for the faculty. Fellowships tend to also be more of an apprenticeship, with longer rotations with faculty. This apprentice-type relationship may be more rewarding to faculty, along with the focus of conferences and research projects in the faculty's own subspecialty area.

Depending on the fellowship, a person's practice postgraduation may in fact be more general orthopaedic surgery rather than their subspecialty choice. For example, the most common fellowship is in the area of sports medicine. The average graduate will join a practice and often do general orthopaedic surgery while building up their subspecialty practice. So, the additional education may not be needed depending on the practice a graduate begins after fellowship.

Do residency graduates need a fellowship? The answer to this question may lie in data from the American Board of

Orthopaedic Surgeons Part II examination results. The ABOS examinations are practice based, and 6 months of procedure log data are submitted to the ABOS within the first 2 years postgraduation. The examination is held after 22 months' postgraduation practice. The exam is based on the individual's collected and submitted cases during this period of time. In a similar manner, orthopaedic surgeons who recertify must submit 6 months of procedure logs with outcomes prior to the recertification examination. The top 15 procedures done for initial Part II examinees and of the recertification examinee (recertification is required to maintain ABOS certification every 8–10 years) are shown in Table 1.1. For the initial examinee, all of the procedures listed come under the purview of general orthopaedic surgery [33]. For those that are recertifying, spine procedures are increased when compared to the initial Part II examinees. So, in practice, the most common procedures do not require subspecialized education of a fellowship.

Defining the scope of capabilities for an orthopaedic surgeon is important for credentialing, board certification, and educational content. Recently, Kellam et al. surveyed practicing general orthopaedic surgeons as part of a General Orthopaedic Competency Task Force (GOCTF) to help determine just what practice skills a general orthopaedic surgeon should have to be safe in practice [33]. The authors described two areas. First, what medical knowledge or office skills should an orthopaedic surgeon have to evaluate a patient and to either treat or refer a patient? Second, what procedures should a general orthopaedic surgeon be capable of performing? The authors compared their results of a survey of 150 practicing "general orthopaedic surgeons" to procedures reported by candidates on the initial Part II Board Certification. The authors found a strong correlation between what a self-identified general orthopaedic surgeon reported to those reported with the Part II examinations. The authors are recommending a content of practice for general orthopaedic surgeons which is the educational goal of an orthopaedic surgery residency program.

Table 1.1 ABOS procedures for 2012

List of the top 15 procedures reported by those who were Part II candidates and those who are MOC diplomates (10 plus years in practice) in 2012

Part II candidates:

29881 Arthroscopy, knee, surgical; with meniscectomy (medial *or* lateral, including any meniscal shaving) including debridement/shaving of articular cartilage (chondroplasty), same or separate compartment(s), when performed

64721 Neuroplasty and/or transposition; median nerve at carpal tunnel

29826 Arthroscopy, shoulder, surgical; decompression of subacromial space with partial acromioplasty, with coracoacromial ligament (i.e., arch) release, when performed

20680 Removal of implant; deep (e.g., buried wire, pin, screw, metal band, nail, rod, or plate)

27447 Arthroplasty, knee, condyle and plateau; medial *and* lateral compartments with or without patella resurfacing (total knee arthroplasty)

29877 Arthroscopy, knee, surgical; debridement/shaving of articular cartilage (chondroplasty)

29888 Arthroscopically aided anterior cruciate ligament repair/ augmentation or reconstruction

27236 Open treatment of femoral fracture, proximal end, neck, internal fixation or prosthetic replacement

11012 Debridement including removal of foreign material at the site of an open fracture and/or an open dislocation (e.g., excisional debridement); skin, subcutaneous tissue, muscle fascia, muscle, and bone for Grade I, II, IIIA and Grade IIIB)

27130 Arthroplasty, acetabular and proximal femoral prosthetic replacement (total hip arthroplasty), with or without autograft or allograft

27245 Treatment of intertrochanteric, peritrochanteric, or subtrochanteric femoral fracture; with intramedullary implant, with or without interlocking screws and/or cerclage

Table 1.1 (continued)

List of the top 15 procedures reported by those who were Part II candidates and those who are MOC diplomates (10 plus years in practice) in 2012

29827 Arthroscopy, shoulder, surgical; with rotator cuff repair

29880 Arthroscopy, knee, surgical; with meniscectomy (medial *and* lateral, including any meniscal shaving) including debridement/shaving of articular cartilage (chondroplasty), same or separate compartment(s), when performed

26055 Tendon sheath incision (e.g., for trigger finger)

27244 Treatment of intertrochanteric, peritrochanteric, or subtrochanteric femoral fracture; with plate/screw type implant, with or without cerclage

MOC diplomats top 15 procedures:

29881 Arthroscopy, knee, surgical; with meniscectomy (medial *or* lateral, including any meniscal shaving) including debridement/shaving of articular cartilage (chondroplasty), same or separate compartment(s), when performed

27447 Arthroplasty, knee, condyle and plateau; medial *and* lateral compartments with or without patella resurfacing (total knee arthroplasty)

29826 Arthroscopy, shoulder, surgical; decompression of subacromial space with partial acromioplasty, with coracoacromial ligament (i.e., arch) release, when performed

29877 Arthroscopy, knee, surgical; debridement/shaving of articular cartilage (chondroplasty)

27130 Arthroplasty, acetabular and proximal femoral prosthetic replacement (total hip arthroplasty), with or without autograft or allograft

64721 Neuroplasty and/or transposition; median nerve at carpal tunnel

29880 Arthroscopy, knee, surgical; with meniscectomy (medial *and* lateral, including any meniscal shaving) including debridement/shaving of articular cartilage (chondroplasty), same or separate compartment(s), when performed

(continued)

TABLE 1.1 (continued)

List of the top 15 procedures reported by those who were Part II candidates and those who are MOC diplomates (10 plus years in practice) in 2012

29827 Arthroscopy, shoulder, surgical; with rotator cuff repair

20680 Removal of implant; deep (e.g., buried wire, pin, screw, metal band, nail, rod, or plate)

29888 Arthroscopically aided anterior cruciate ligament repair/ augmentation or reconstruction

29824 Arthroscopy, shoulder, surgical; distal claviculectomy including distal articular surface (Mumford procedure)

63047 Laminectomy, facetectomy, and foraminotomy (unilateral or bilateral with decompression of spinal cord, cauda equina, and/or nerve root[s] [e.g., spinal or lateral recess stenosis]), single vertebral segment; lumbar

26055 Tendon sheath incision (e.g., for trigger finger)

22612 Arthrodesis, posterior or posterolateral technique, single level; lumbar (with lateral transverse technique, when performed)

29823 Arthroscopy, shoulder, surgical; debridement, extensive

The 12th edition of *Campbell's Operative Orthopaedics* was published in 2012, with 4664 pages of content for the four-volume set. While including refinements and increased electronic media, as well as an electronic version, the content had not changed over the preceding two editions when reviewing those topics of a general orthopaedic surgeon.

Summary

Orthopaedic surgery residency education has evolved since the early twentieth century to its present state of providing high-quality operative surgeons to care for the public. At the time of this writing, orthopaedic surgery residency programs have undergone major structural changes over the past 3 years. It remains to be seen how the NAS, intern surgical skills, and resident duty hours have affected resident education. Education should be based on what the future needs of the population might be, providing doctors who are skilled to treat that population. In doing so, future planning should be oriented towards establishing a cohesive educational structure and content for orthopaedic surgery of the future, and building education towards serving that goal.

References

1. Johns Hopkins Orthopaedic Surgery Department. History. See http://www.hopkinsmedicine.org/orthopaedic-surgery/about-us/dept-history.html. Accessed February 20, 2017.
2. HerndonJ. Osgood lecture. Harv Orthopaed J. http://www.orthojournalhms.org/volume11/thesisday/index.htm. Accessed February 20, 2017.
3. American Board of Orthopaedic Surgeons. Rules and procedures. 1936.
4. American Board of Orthopaedic Surgeons. Rules and procedures. 1943.
5. Shands AR. Conference on post graduate education in orthopaedic surgery. J Bone Joint Surg. 1949;31A:887–8.
6. Campbell WC. Operative orthopaedics. St Louis: CV Mosby; 1939.
7. Azar FM, Beaty JH, editors. Campbell's operative orthopaedics. 13th ed. Philadelphia: Elsevier Health Sciences; 2016.
8. Speed JS, SmithH. Campbell's operative orthopaedics, 2. (2 vols) CV Mosby, St Louis. 1949.
9. Street D. Resident training in a veterans administration hospital. J Bone Joint Surg. 1949;31A:895–6.
10. Green WT. The ideal curriculum in children's orthopaedic surgery. JBJS. 1949;31A:889–90.
11. Speed JS, Knight RA (ed). Campbell's operative orthopaedics, 2. (2 vols) CV Mosby, St Louis. 1956.
12. Luck JV. Orthopaedic surgery-shaping it for permanence or ending? J Bone Joint Surg. 1962;44A:390–7.
13. Robinson RA. Ideal preparation for academic orthopaedics. J Bone Joint Surg. 1961;43A:789–90.
14. Crenshaw AW (ed) Campbell's operative orthopaedics, 2. (2 vols) CV Mosby, St Louis, 1963.

15. Mankin HK, Carter RM, Krawczyk A. The effect of permissive environment on scoring of the orthopaedic in-training examination. J Bone Joint Surg Am. 1973;55A:1100–11.
16. Dougherty PJ, Walter N, Schilling P, Najibi S, Herkowitz H. Do scores of the USMLE step 1 and OITE correlate with the ABOS part I certifying examination? Clin Orthop Rel Res. 2010;468:2797–802.
17. Wilson PD. All for one, one for all. J Bone Joint Surg. 1973;55A:859–965.
18. EdmonsonAS, CrenshawAH. Campbell's operative orthopaedics, 6. (2 vols). CV Mosby, St Louis, 1980.
19. Enneking WF. The education of future orthopaedists. J Bone Joint Surg. 1984;66A:1139–42.
20. Gregory CF. Wither orthopaedics? Circa 1973. J Bone Joint Surg. 1973;55A:1537–43.
21. CrenshawAH (ed). Speed JS, SmithH. Campbell's operative orthopaedics, 2. (5 vols) CV Mosby, St Louis 1992.
22. Kohn LT, Corrigan JM, Donaldson MS, editors. To err is human: building a safer health system. Washington, DC: Institute of Medicine; 1999.
23. Ludmerer K. Let me heal. Oxford: Oxford University Press; 2014.
24. Bohm KC, Hill BW, Braman JP, Ly TV, Van Heest AE. Orthopedic residency: are duty hours predictive of performance? J Surg Educ. 2016;73:281–5.
25. Dougherty PJ. What the ACGME's next accreditation System means to you. Clin Orthop Relat Res. 2013;479:2746–50.
26. Dougherty PJ, Marcus RE. ACGME and ABOS changes for the orthopaedic surgery PGY-1 (intern) year. Clin Orthop Relat Res. 2013; 471:3412–6.
27. Weiss KB, Bagian JP, Wagner R. CLER pathways to excellence. Expectations for a clinical learning environment. J Grad Med Educ. 2014:610–1.
28. Carter PR. The embryogenesis of the specialty of hand surgery: a story of three great Americans—a politician, a general, and a duck hunter: the 2002 Richard J. Smith memorial lecture. J Hand Surg Am. 2003;28:185–98.
29. Simon MA. Evolution of the status of orthopaedic surgery fellowships. J Bone Joint Surg Am. 1998;80A:1826–9.
30. Cooper RC. Impact of fellowships on orthopaedic surgery residencies,patient care, and orthopaedic practice. Part I. J Bone Joint Surg Am. 1998;80A:1829–30.

31. Urbaniak JR. Impact of fellowships on orthopaedic surgery residencies,patient care, and orthopaedic practice. Part II. J Bone Joint Surg Am. 1998;80A:1830–3.
32. Horst PK, Choo K, Bharucha N, Vail TP. Topics in training. Graduates of orthopaedic residency trainingare increasingly subspecialized. A review of the American Board of Orthopaedic Surgery. Part II database J. Bone Joint Surg Am. 2015;97:869–75.
33. Kellam JF, Archibald D, Barber JW, Christian EP, D'Ascoli RJ, Haynes RJ, Hecht SS, Hurwitz SR, Kellam JF, McLaren AC, Peabody TD, Southworth SR, Strauss RW, Wadey VM. The Core competencies for general orthopaedic surgeons. J Bone Joint Surg Am. 2017;99:175–81.

Chapter 2
Orthopaedic Education in Other Countries

Paul J. Dougherty

Introduction

Orthopaedic education in other countries around the world shows a rich variation in how education is provided. The purpose of any graduate medical education program is to provide competent practitioners who will meet the needs of the country. The three countries described here, India, the UK, and Germany, provide a glimpse of how the structure of graduate medical education has recently changed to meet the needs of both patients and the individual learners (Fig. 2.1) [1–3].

This chapter hopes to explore how orthopaedic residencies are presently organized in each country, what recent changes have occurred, and what are the strengths and weaknesses of each country's programs.

P.J. Dougherty, MD
Department of Orthopaedic Surgery, University of Florida College of Medicine—Jacksonville, 655 W 8th Street, 2nd Floor ACC, Jacksonville, FL 32209, USA
e-mail: paul.dougherty@jax.ufl.edu

© Springer International Publishing AG 2018
P.J. Dougherty, B.L. Joyce (eds.), *The Orthopedic Educator*,
DOI 10.1007/978-3-319-62944-5_2

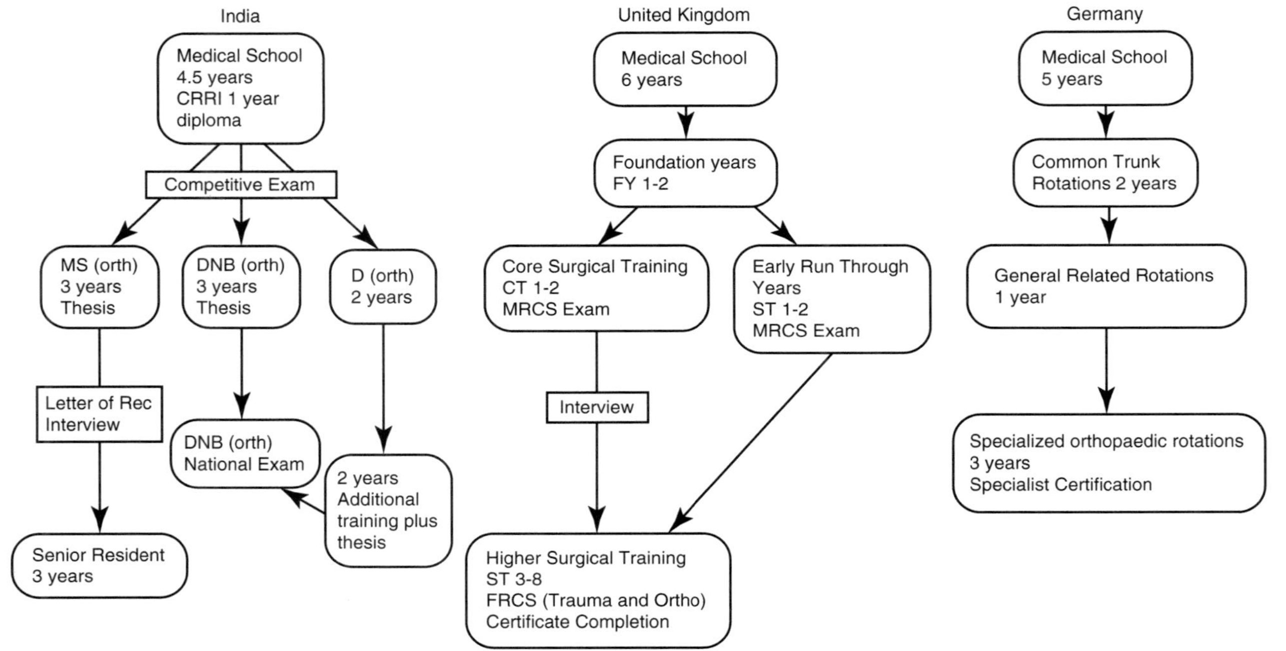

FIGURE 2.1 Orthopaedic education in India, the UK, and Germany

India

India is the second most populous country in the world, 1.25 billion in 2013, with a very diverse economy and somewhat differing medical burden than is seen in Western Europe and the United States. There are also less doctors in India, 0.7/1000 population versus the 2.45/1000 seen in the United States [4]. Because of poverty, the burden from infectious disease remains relatively higher than in Western countries [5, 6]. Safe drinking water remains a problem for a large segment of the population. Tuberculosis remains prevalent in India [5, 6]. That said, there have been tremendous strides over the last 50 years to decrease this disease burden. Because of improvements in public health, there has been an increasing proportion of the population deaths attributed to trauma rather than infectious disease [5]. The practice of orthopaedic surgery has also changed. Orthopaedic surgery practice still continues to be largely for the treatment of trauma and infections, but steadier progress has been made for a segment of the population to have care available for elective spine, adult reconstruction, and sports diagnoses [1, 5]. Therefore, the practice of orthopaedic surgery is slowly infusing more sophisticated (and expensive) care commonly seen in Europe and the United States.

Medical College

Unlike the United States, students in India enter medical school after graduating high school. The criterion for admission into medical school is based upon a national written examination. India has a large number of schools and applications. Because of this, the single written examination is generally the criteria for admission [1, 6].

Upon completion of medical school, students earn a Bachelor of Medicine and Bachelor of Surgery (MBBS) degree. Following completion of basic medical training, students enter a 1-year Compulsory Rotating Residential Internship (CRRI).

This program is similar to a rotating or transitional internship. Upon successful completion of the CRRI, medical students receive medical college diplomas [1, 6].

Medical school candidates are exposed to a wide variety of specialty areas that serve the needs of the country prior to making their selection of career. This differs from the American experience, in which a medical student generally applies for specialty training at the end of their third year in medical school.

In order to apply for residency specialty training, MBBS graduates must pass a national-level and/or state-level "post-graduate entrance exam"—a written exam that is the deciding factor for placement in postgraduate training.

Residency

Basic Surgical Education

Currently, residents in India can obtain orthopaedic surgery education via three main pathways: a university-based Masters (MS Orthopaedics) program, a Diplomate of National Board (DNB) program, and a Diploma in Orthopaedic Surgery (D.Ortho) program [1, 5, 6, 7].

Residents can earn a Master of Surgery degree in orthopaedic surgery, MS (Orthopaedics), upon successful completion of a 3-year orthopaedic specialty training program. In order to gain eligibility for an exit examination, residents must pass the standard national curriculum for resident exposure and education, and successfully complete a required thesis. The curriculum covers all aspects of general orthopaedic surgery, including pathology (which itself deals with conditions especially common in India, in particular infections and tuberculosis). According to the Medical Council of India, there are 225 MS (Orthopaedics) training programs available to residents. For the 2012–2013 years, 919 slots were available for the first-year postgraduate orthopaedic class [8]. That number is quite small when considering the population of the country. Just what the "right number" might be is hard to discern when considering the size and scope of the entire Indian health system.

Like other countries, orthopaedic surgery is a popular specialty for postmedical school education, and the need for further specialists is warranted. Candidates who fail to earn admission into the MS programs can also apply for the 3-year Diplomate of National Board (DNB) program in nonuniversity-affiliated hospitals. In order to gain enrollment in DNB courses, MBBS students must take a national-level common entrance examination conducted by National Board of Examination. D.Orth candidates who wrote a thesis and have 2 additional years of education may also be eligible to take the DNB exams. Qualified MS (Orthopaedics) candidates may take the exit examination for DNB without any further training. The course structure is on par with the Medical Council of India's recognized courses [1].

Recognizing the overwhelming interest in obtaining a MS (Orthopaedics) degree, the Medical Council of India supervises another pathway for entrance into orthopaedics called the Diploma in Orthopaedic Surgery (D.Orth) program. In 2013, the 2-year D.Orth program offered 110 courses with 309 first-year seats available. This program is to provide graduates who will provide care in areas of limited resources with a more limited scope than seen with the 3-year curriculum.

Senior Education

Further training as a senior resident in orthopaedic surgery is available in few select states/universities/hospitals. Senior resident training runs for a further 3 years, and is less structured than the MS education. The senior resident will care for patients along with faculty members at their hospital. The senior resident is also given more autonomy to run their own operating room and clinic, with indirect supervision of a faculty member. Admission for a senior residency is based on recommendations and interviews. Each institution is slightly different, but generally, it takes 3 calendar years to complete a senior residency. There are even fewer senior resident positions available than those at the MS-level program. Therefore, not all Masters graduates will receive further training.

Candidates who did not succeed in obtaining a senior resident position are also deemed to be orthopaedic surgeons and are authorized to practice the specialty. However due to their insufficient surgical experience many will opt for a junior staff position under the indirect guidance of a senior surgeon. Others may work in a less served area practicing office orthopaedics and a few basic surgical procedures [1, 5].

Fellowship training, beyond Senior Residency, is offered by the National Board of Examinations in hand and microvascular surgery, spine, and trauma. These 2-year fellowships are available postgraduation, but usually have no more than ten spots available for the entire country [1, 5].

Strengths

There are a number of strengths to Indian orthopaedic medical education. Senior orthopaedic residents work in a more traditional model. They will run their own operating room while in the supervision of a consultant. This allows for autonomy and developing surgical skills in a safe environment. As a senior resident's skills progress, he or she is given more autonomy. Under this system, the senior resident must demonstrate the ability to care independently for patients.

The Indian medical education is provided in English, and both junior and senior residents are exposed to the world's leading medical journals for orthopaedic surgery. Additionally, textbooks are printed in English, allowing for a broad exposure to world orthopaedic surgery. Since (MS Orthopaedics) training is provided in high-patient-population institutions, the trainee learns how to utilize his or her basic skills in decision making and handling large patient loads.

Although tuberculosis and polio are not commonly found in the United States, Indian orthopaedic education emphasizes these diseases, as well as neglected fractures and clubfoot. Caring for these diagnoses serves the needs of the country's patient population [5, 6].

Limitations

As orthopaedic care in India has become more complex, Indian orthopaedic surgeons have noted that the Masters-level training in India is not comprehensive enough, and some graduates may have insufficient training to practice independently. Future modifications should include a longer residency program (possibly adding 1–2 years of mandatory education), and create mechanisms (such as board certification processes) that ensure physician competence. Furthermore, emphasis on preparing graduates to care for common problems in India, such as tuberculosis or neglected fractures, could be improved. These further educational opportunities for MS/DNB graduates must be readily available [5, 6].

Conclusion

Given the relative shortage of doctors to the population, the limited resources available to care for patients, and the wide variety of diagnoses orthopaedic surgeons are expected to treat, Indian education has made tremendous strides to provide the best for the most people.

UK

The UK includes a population of 64.1 million people (2013) within its borders. There is an abundance of physicians in the UK (2.81/1000 population) vs. the United States (2.45/1000 population) [2, 4]. Healthcare in the UK is largely provided by the National Healthcare Service (NHS) which also provides the financing of graduate medical education. Graduate medical education in the UK recently restructured with the goal of improving trainee experience. In 2005, the Modernizing Medical Careers program changed the organizational structure of all postmedical school training in the UK due to concerns about excess length of training and a lack of supervision [8]. The goals were to include standardization of education and training to produce "high-quality, well-trained, accredited doctors." A more formalized structure of feedback and assessment has also been implemented to document the progress of trainees [8]. Additionally, the European Union's European Work Time Directive (EWTD) reduced the number of hours any employee could work (including those in graduate medical education training)—from 56 to 48 h per week [9].

Orthopaedic Training: The Foundation Years

Medical school is a 5-year program, beginning after secondary (high) school. Graduates obtain a "Bachelor of Medicine, Bachelor of Surgery" which is abbreviated in a variety of ways (MB BS, BM BCh, MB BCh, MB BCh BAO, etc.), depending on the institution. All are equivalent degrees, which allow the graduate to be qualified for further education.

Orthopaedic registrar education is divided into three phases: the "foundation years," core surgical training, and then higher surgical training. In the foundation years (FY1–2), the new physician obtains further education regarding basic patient care skills. These years (Fig. 2.1) are similar to an internship in the United States, with exposure to different medical areas, providing broad exposure to other medical conditions. During the first 2 years, the trainee is eligible to take Part A of the Member Royal College of Surgeons exam.

Orthopaedic education in the UK is described as Trauma and Orthopaedic (Tr & Orth), recognizing the need to care for patients who have sustained trauma, and the large dependency on the healthcare system to care for patients with fractures [10].

Core Specialty Education

The next level of training, called core specialty training (CT1 and CT2), is appointed by competitive interview. Core specialty training begins after the foundation years, and is considered the initial surgical specialty training. There are run-through programs, in which the candidate progresses directly to the later years of surgical training. Those who are in run-through programs are designated as specialty trainees (ST) instead of CT1 and CT2. Specialty trainees may rotate in no more than two related surgical fields for up to 6 months each. The first year (CT1 or ST1) focuses on the care of trauma patients, the management of simple fractures, and principles of both internal and external fixation. The second year, CT2/ST2, builds on the previous year, developing more extensive surgical skills for fracture fixation (intra-articular, open, and hip fractures for example), and initial exposure to elective types of procedures. During the second year, the trainee is eligible to take Part B of the Member Royal College of Surgeons exam, consisting of a patient-based simulation exam (objective structured clinical exam) [12].

Alternate Pathway if Unsuccessful Core Training

At the end of CT2, trainees who have been unsuccessful in passing the Member Royal College of Surgeons exam or who have not gained a National Training Number for ST3–8 training may apply for a further year in core training for experience, undertake a clinical fellowship (junior posts which do not have official recognition for training), or apply for a Specialty Doctor/Non-Consultant Hospital Doctor post. Specialty Doctor posts are permanent subconsultant career posts. Doctors who have worked in these posts for several years can apply to the General Medical Council for Specialist registration if they have equivalent experience to a day 1 Consultant, and have passed the Fellow of the Royal

College of Surgeons (FRCS) (Tr & Orth) examination. This, however, is a lengthy process and the award is by no means automatic [12].

Higher Surgical Training

Appointment to a Higher Surgical Training post (ST3–8) is by competitive interview. Scotland and England run a competitive single-center multi-station interview. Wales and Northern Ireland each run their own multi-station interviews. The job specification is centrally determined by the Orthopaedic Specialist Advisory Committee and ratified by Health Education England. In England, the number of posts is set by the Centre for Workforce Intelligence, which may not reflect the needs of the specialty. The devolved regions are able to set their own recruitment numbers. In any given year, between 120 and 150 ST3s will be appointed. There are generally between five and ten applicants for each post [14, 15].

At the end of the intermediate years, considered ST3–6, the trainee gains experience with various subspecialties, such as foot and ankle, hip, knee, shoulder/elbow, and hand. Rotations are structured for 6 months in length, and may be at other institutions than the main teaching hospital [15].

After ST6, 2 additional years of training (ST7–8) are conducted to further refine the skills in general orthopaedic surgery and trauma, along with additional clinical training in a specialty area [8, 10]. The trainee is now eligible to take the examination to become a FRCS (Tr and Orth). Trainees should have a minimum of 1800 cases recorded in their logbooks (assisted and performed), encompassing the generality of Trauma and Orthopaedic Surgery by the end of ST6. They are also expected to perform at least 12 index procedures. Trainees must show evidence of undertaking one audit each year, including two completed audit cycles. They are also expected to present two research presentations at national meetings and publish two peer-reviewed publications. Trainees may undertake full-time research during their training, but will only gain 6 months' recognition for this, regardless of the time in research. The recognition of time spent in research is conditional on successful completion of a research degree or publication of the results of research [2, 8, 10].

Upon completion of the 6-year Higher Surgical Training program, a trainee applies to the Joint Committee on Surgical Training for a Completion of Training certification. When this is awarded, the trainee is enrolled on the Specialist Register of the General Medical Council as an Orthopaedic Specialist. This entitles the trainee to practice as an orthopaedic specialist in any European Union member state. At this stage, most trainees elect to undertake a further period of fellowship training in their chosen subspecialty [2, 8, 10].

Strengths

As it is presently constituted, orthopaedic training takes place within a clear framework, defining what is expected of the trainee, trainer, and training program [10–12]. The trainee portfolio provides clear and detailed evidence of a trainee's progress against defined standards, and helps to distinguish between successful and failing trainees. The latter can be identified, and targeted training can be instituted. The relationship between trainer and trainee requires a significant investment in time and effort but delivers a clearer understanding of what is needed for training [2, 10–12].

For a program director, guidelines help confirm that training posts are appropriate for trainees and ensure that provision of training is considered by medical management.

Limitations

While it is unclear just what effect the EWTD has had on orthopaedic education, it is felt that with the increasing complexity of the field and the decreased amount of time available for work, educational programs will need to be made longer [10, 13, 17, 18].

Prior to the Modernizing Medical Careers program, more autonomy was possible for the trainee to run their own "list" of operating room. Less challenging cases could be performed independently, with indirect supervision of a consultant (faculty or fully trained supervisor). More challenging cases would have help readily available.

While having clear guidelines is helpful, setting specified numerical targets in 12 index operations is a skewing surgical experience. What started as a competency-based training program, allowing each trainee to develop skills at different rates, has now become driven by quantity. Good trainees are diverted from gaining a breadth of surgical experience by focusing on "getting their numbers" [11, 16].

A further impediment to a trainee's surgical experience is the widespread use of the independent sector for provision of elective orthopaedic surgery. In order to meet waiting time targets, the National Health Service transfers patients to the private sector for surgery. These are often more straightforward cases, which would be ideal for training, but are lost to the pool of training.

Germany

There is a high physician density within Germany, 3.89/1000 population, when compared to the United States (2.45/1000 population) [4]. This makes the practice of medicine one of the most competitive in the world.

Although education in Germany is free to the student, there is a high competition to get into certain fields, with medicine the most competitive—only about 5% of the top students will get admitted, based on grades, or a combination of grades and/or the results of a specialized test for medicine. Medical school in Germany generally takes a minimum of 6 years to complete. The first 2 years are equivalent to a college education, consisting of topics such as physics, chemistry, and biochemistry. The second part of medical school is almost purely clinical, consisting of rotations in internal medicine, general or orthopaedic surgery, and a 4-month rotation of the student's choice. The sixth year is similar to a general rotating internship in the United States, after which the new graduate (usually about 24 years of age) is eligible for medical licensure in a similar manner to an internship graduate in the United States [19].

Residency

Historically in Germany, postgraduate orthopaedic surgery education was surgery based, with 6 years of general surgery the basis of any kind of further subspecialization (cardiovascular, thoracic, plastics, trauma, etc.). Along with the developments of the AO (Arbeitsgemeinschaft Osteosynthese, ASIF) starting in 1958, the orthopaedic trauma subspecialization began to develop and there was a dramatic increase in the surgical case load for fracture, most importantly because suddenly techniques became available to stabilize all kinds of truncal and extremity injuries. This generated the identification of another subspecialty, the Unfallchirurg. This expert was expected to be able to take care of all injuries, including the surgical fracture care. The Unfallchirurg would be a surgeon who in the United States today would have the expertise of orthopaedic trauma, general surgery, and acute care surgery [2, 20].

German orthopaedic surgery postgraduate training changed from "orthopaedics and traumatology" to orthopaedic surgery in 2003 to match similar educational residency programs in the European Union (Fig. 2.1). This was done for two main reasons. First, by 2003, medical educators believed that 6 years of preliminary general surgery education was excessive, leading to longer postgraduate training plus education in areas not commonly practiced by an orthopaedic surgeon. The US and other systems served as a template as well, allowing for more focused education covering a broad spectrum of orthopaedic surgery. Second, leaders from German residency training programs realized that standardization of training in Europe would allow for easier migration within the European Union. More importantly, a standardized curriculum allows for more consistent education and postgraduation performance. The move to a more uniform, streamlined, and focused educational residency program led to a decrease in government costs and allowed for more potential years as a practicing surgeon [20–23].

German orthopaedic residency takes about 6 years to complete. There are two initial years of "common trunk rotations" which expose the resident to different specialties, much like a surgical internship. These rotations are similar for a number of specialties. Following this, there is a year of "general related rotations" which are more specific to the field of orthopaedic surgery, followed by another 3 years of orthopaedic specific education [2, 20–22].

This new structure for German orthopaedic surgery residency is a large departure from the previous educational experience. German doctors ultimately spend less time in training to become practicing orthopaedic surgeons (from 11 to 6 years total). That being said, the new residency model is more consistent with programs seen in other countries and the European Union. It is hard to assess how well these changes help produce better doctors when compared to other countries, and there is not a "universal formula for the best residency program," although a Europe-wide respected board of trauma surgery qualification exists (the European Board of Surgery Qualification [EBSQ]). The EBSQ is a standardized exam that consists of an oral exam, a written test, and an exam to assess the ability to speak and understand the English language. It is held annually during the German Orthopaedic meeting and in association with the European Society of Trauma and Emergency Surgery [20].

Another change is the new German residency structure that allows for the program Chairman to determine when the resident is actually ready to graduate, as opposed to a resident completing the program based only on strict time guidelines. This allows for more time in training to develop skills at an individual's pace. As residency programs tend to be smaller (2–3 per year group), the ability to provide more individual education throughout the residency is a benefit. Future initiatives, in which the resident rotations become more focused in both content and assessment, are being discussed by German orthopaedic educators. This trend is also occurring in other countries. With US residency programs, the decision to delay graduation based on performance is more difficult because of the perception that residency is complete when the 5 years of residency is complete. Knowing that variation occurs with student abilities makes this "one-size-fits-all" standard unlikely.

German Fellowships

A fellowship for elective orthopaedic surgery (arthroplasty) or orthopaedic trauma generally follows training. There are prerequisites for those that chose to work in a certified arthroplasty unit or a Level 1 trauma center. Further specialization in either "specialized trauma surgery" or "specialized orthopaedic surgery" requires another 2 to 3 years of training. "Specialized trauma surgery" requires an additional 420 surgical cases [21–22].

Other fellowships do exist in Germany, but differ in structure and content from those in other countries. There are "extra qualifications" (*"zusatz weiterbildung"*) in "special orthopaedic surgery" which are an additional 36 months' education. In the United States, orthopaedic fellowships are generally 1 year in length.

Limitations

Both faculty and those in training have raised concerns that there is insufficient time for certain rotations to provide continuity of care or sufficient surgical volume, though recent documentation shows that residents can document adequate case volumes. The European Working Time Directive officially allows for a total 48 h of in-house service per week.

The application of the European Working Time Directive has been slow to occur, and residency training programs across the European Union were initially given several years to phase in the work-hour restrictions. Concerns regarding the rigid time directives still remain, and some flexibility in these rules for those in training to assure adequate breadth of experience will still need to be discussed [2, 21, 25].

To put the work-hour restrictions in perspective, Luring et al. surveyed orthopaedic training programs in Germany to determine how many of the procedures were performed by trainees as opposed to faculty [24]. For 35,654 knee arthroscopies, 49% were performed by senior surgeons, 28% by junior attendings, and 27% by trainees. Of 30,642 shoulder arthroscopies, the percentages were 78%, 18%, and 7%, respectively. Of 31,138 knee arthroplasties, the respective percentages were 80%, 14%, and 7%. The authors concluded that there are opportunities to improve the hands-on experience of those in training.

Researchers conducted a survey of academic Orthopaedic Chiefs or *"Chefarzten"* from the German Society of Trauma and the German Society of Orthopaedic Surgery to assess their perception of the capabilities of new graduates ("new specialist") in clinical knowledge and patient care [20]. A survey sent to 954 (220 respondents) Chairmen (Chefarzte/Chefarztinnen) showed a perception of limited competence for the graduates. Respondents felt that only 52% of new graduates could handle standard surgical approaches to large joints, and only 24% could independently conduct standard surgical procedures. A recent survey voted against a reduction of the minimum number of surgical cases required by graduates, and are interested in keeping the specialty primarily operative in nature. Additionally, the survey also reported that 86% of those surveyed felt that surgery should be done by the residents themselves, with appropriate supervision. This concern about graduates being ready to practice is found in other countries. For example, a recent survey of orthopaedic program directors in the United

States found that only 17% agreed that all graduates were ready to be attending surgeons.

Conclusion

These three examples are of how individual nations meet their orthopaedic education needs. Graduate medical education in all three countries is done to provide a sufficient supply of trained orthopaedic surgeons who can care for the population.

Indian orthopaedic education is designed to produce competent practitioners through various pathways, allowing for a needed volume of orthopaedic surgeons with various skill levels with 2- and 3-year programs, with a select few going on to have senior resident education. Because of higher workloads, residents get autonomy as they demonstrate competence in certain clinical areas. This allows for demonstration of being able to independently practice before the completion of the educational process.

In Europe, changes with the EWTD have placed constraints on the ability to provide sufficient clinical experience within the allotted amount of time for residency has led to discussion about extending the time in training. Additional changes seen in both the UK and Germany has been a more focused training program. In the UK, education has become shortened and more prescribed, without being a registrar for several years. In Germany, the elimination of the general surgical education prior to orthopaedic surgery-specific training has led to a shortening of the basic orthopaedic education in that country.

Finally, educators in all countries recognize the gradual increase in the complexity of the specialty. In all examples, there has been a trend to streamline the education, as well as discussion about increasing the amount of training needed to be proficient in the specialty.

References

1. Dougherty PJ, Sethi A, Jain AK. Orthopaedic surgery education in India. Clin Orthop Relat Res. 2014;472(2):410–4.
2. McAlinden MG, Dougherty PJ. Orthopaedic education in the United Kingdom. Clin Orthop Relat Res. 2014;472:1697–702.
3. Pape HC, Dougherty PJ. CORR (®) curriculum—orthopaedic education: the evolution of orthopaedic surgery education in Germany. Clin Orthop Relat Res. 2015;473:2464–8.
4. CIA World Fact Book. https://www.cia.gov/library/publications/the-world-factbook/fields/2226.html Accessed Nov 7, 2016.
5. Jain AK. Current state of orthopedic education in India. Indian J Orthop. 2016;50(4):341–4.
6. Arora A, Agarwal A, Gikas P, Mehra A. Musculoskeletal training for orthopaedists and nonorthopaedists: experiences in India. Clin Orthop Relat Res. 2008;466:2350–9.
7. The Medical Council of India. http://www.mciindia.org. Accessed Nov 7, 2016.
8. House of Commons Health Committee. Modernizing medical careers, vol. 2. Written evidence. http://www.parliament.the-stationery-office.co.uk/pa/cm200708/cmselect/cmhealth/25/25ii.pdf. Accessed Feb 24, 2014.
9. Tooke J, Ashtinany S, Carter D, Cole A, Michael J, Rashid A, Smith PC, Tomlinson S, Petty-Saphon K. Aspiring to excellence. The final report of the independent inquiry into modernizing medical careers. Chiswick: Aldridge Press; 2008. p. 1–238.
10. Invaparthy P, Sayana M, Maffuli M. Evolving trauma and orthopaedics training in the UK. J Surg Ed. 2013;70:104–8.
11. Joint Committee on Surgical Training. Guidelines for the award of CCT in Trauma and Orthopaedic Surgery. http://www.jcst.org/quality_assurance/Docs/cct_guidelines_to. Accessed Jan 10, 2014.
12. British Orthopaedic Association. The surgical pathway. http://www.boa.ac.uk/training-education/the-surgical-training-process/ Accessed Nov 7, 2016.
13. Centre for Workforce Intelligence. Medical Specialty Workforce Factsheet. Trauma and orthopaedic surgery. http://www.cfwi.org.uk/publications/trauma-and-orthopaedic-surgery-cfwi-medical-fact-sheet-and-summary-sheet-august-2011. Accessed Nov 11, 2016.
14. General Medical Council. http://www.gmc-uk.org/doctors/statistics.asp. Accessed Jan 20, 2014.

15. Frostick S, Baird E, Bale S, et al. Specialist training in trauma and orthopaedics. Curriculum August 2013. London: British Orthopaedic Association, Royal College of Surgeons; 2013.
16. Pitts D, Rowley D, Sher L. Assessment of performance in orthopaedic training. J Bone Joint Surg Br. 2005;87:1187–991.
17. Marron CD, Byrnes CK, Kirk SJ. An EWTD compliant shift rotation decreases SHO training opportunities. Ann R Coll Surg Engl. 2005;87(Suppl):246–8.
18. Wilson T, Sahu A, Johnson DS, Truner PG. The effect of trainee involvement on procedure and list times: a statistical analysis with discussion of current issues affecting orthopaedic training in UK. Surgeon. 2010;8:15–9.
19. Chenot JF. Undergraduate medical education in Germany [in German]. Ger Med Sci. 2009;7:2.
20. Niethard M, Depeweg D. 6 years after reformation of the specialty training reglementation—is there still room for improvement? [in German]. Z Orthop Unfall. 2010;148:471–5.
21. Chances and risks of a new residency program for orthopedics and trauma surgery [in German]. Z Orthop Unfall. 2013;151:126–8.
22. Achatz G, Perl M, Stange R, Mutschler M, Jarvers JS, Münzberg M. How many generalists and how many specialists does orthopedics and traumatology need? [in German]. Unfallchirg. 2013;116:29–33.
23. Pape HC. Restricted duty hours and implications on resident education-are different trauma systems effected in a different way? Injury. 2010;41:125–7.
24. Luring C, Tingart M, Beckmann J, Grifka J, Bathis H. Surgical training in orthopaedic and trauma departments in Germany [in German]. Z Orthop Unfall. 2010;148:466–70.
25. Mauser NS, Michelson JD, Gissel H, Henderson C, Mauffrey C. Work-hour restrictions and orthopaedic resident education: a systematic review. Int Orthop. 2016;40(5):865–73.

Chapter 3
Curriculum Design for Competency-Based Education in Orthopaedics

Barbara L. Joyce and Kathleen McHale

Background of Competency-Based Education

External factors, such as increasing public and governmental pressure to train competent physicians, prompted the Accreditation Council of Graduate Medical Education (ACGME) and American Board of Medical Specialties (ABMS) in 1999 to introduce a model of competency-based education for physician training and certification. The ACGME and ABMS identified the following competency domains: Medical Knowledge (MK), Patient Care (PC), Interpersonal and Communication Skills (ICS), Professionalism (P), Systems-based Practice (SBP), and Practice-based Learning and Improvement (PBLI) [1].

B.L. Joyce, PhD (✉)
Oakland University William Beaumont School of Medicine,
446 O'Dowd Hall, 2200 N. Squirrel Road,
Rochester, MI 48307, USA
e-mail: joyce@oakland.edu

K. McHale, MD, MSEd
George Washington University, Uniformed Services
University for the Health Sciences, 6004 Bitternut Drive,
Alexandria, VA 22130, USA
e-mail: colmchale@yahoo.com

© Springer International Publishing AG 2018
P.J. Dougherty, B.L. Joyce (eds.), *The Orthopedic Educator*,
DOI 10.1007/978-3-319-62944-5_3

Moving from a process and structure model of training to a competency-based model of training produced a transformational shift in physician training. Residency training programs had to redesign curricula, develop more robust assessment tools, improve training through the use of continuous improvement techniques, and create a greater curricular focus on topics such as quality and safety, communication skills, and professionalism. This large-scale initiative was named the Outcome Project, as a means of highlighting the importance of educational outcomes in physician training [2].

Competency-based medical education (CBME) is an educational approach that utilizes domains of competence and their educational outcomes as an overarching framework for training [3–5]. Competency domains encompass broad domains of knowledge, skills, and attitudes [1, 2]. Each competency domain is further delineated into specific sub-competencies which specify the knowledge, skills, and attitudes trainees should acquire within each larger competency domain [1, 2]. The ACGME phased in accreditation requirements requiring that all graduate medical education (GME) training programs develop competency-based curricula, as well as, identify the educational outcomes of training. The background and training of the traditional surgeon educator have been devoid of education theory—the basics of teaching and evaluation. Consequently, many programs struggled to redesign curricula in attempts to meet accreditation requirements, and were unable to identify educational outcomes. For many, the competencies were too abstract, and did not provide a clear-cut way to identify appropriate assessment methods or tools. Metrics at the individual and the program levels were deficient or misdirected. Swing (2007) acknowledged that the paradigm shift to competency-based education was arduous for graduate medical education, but stated that progress had been made in expanding perceptions about physician competence, as well as expanding the field's understanding of how to best assess trainees [2]. The ACGME/ABMS competencies reflected early attempts at providing a common language and framework for competency-based

GME, but fell short in providing robust educational outcomes at the individual and program levels [2].

In 2013, the ACGME introduced the Milestone Project [6]. The milestones were designed to define benchmarks of resident achievement for each of the sub-competencies. Ideally, the milestones assist the trainee with charting a course of learning and will provide faculty with key benchmarks the resident should achieve during training. The milestones were organized along a developmental continuum from novice to expert, which reflected increasing professional competence [6, 7]. Individual resident performance data can be aggregated to form a snapshot of program performance on each of the milestones. Clinical Competency Committees were formed to determine each resident's performance on the milestones based on aggregate assessment data [6]. More recently, Entrustable Professional Activities (EPAs) have been introduced in some specialties, such as Internal Medicine and Pediatrics, but have not yet been introduced in Orthopaedic Surgery (at the time of writing this chapter) [8–10]. "EPAs are those professional activities that together constitute the mass of critical elements that operationally define a profession" [10, p. 544]. EPAs reflect routine activities of physicians, whereas competencies describe abilities at a particular point in training or in a specific context [11]. Please see Fig. 3.1 for a hierarchical depiction of EPAs, competencies, sub-competencies, and milestones (Fig. 3.1).

Orthopaedic Surgery was one of the initial seven specialties to adopt milestones as a framework for resident assessment. Workgroups, consisting of experts in orthopaedic surgery, identified 16 milestones, based on key surgical procedures in orthopaedic surgery. The milestones were reflective of knowledge and skill in Medical Knowledge and Patient Care [11]. In addition, an additional nine milestones were written for four of the generic core competencies (P, ICS, PBLI, and SBP). However, the orthopaedic surgery milestones have not been outlined for the entire six domains of competence and sub-competencies required for completion of training.

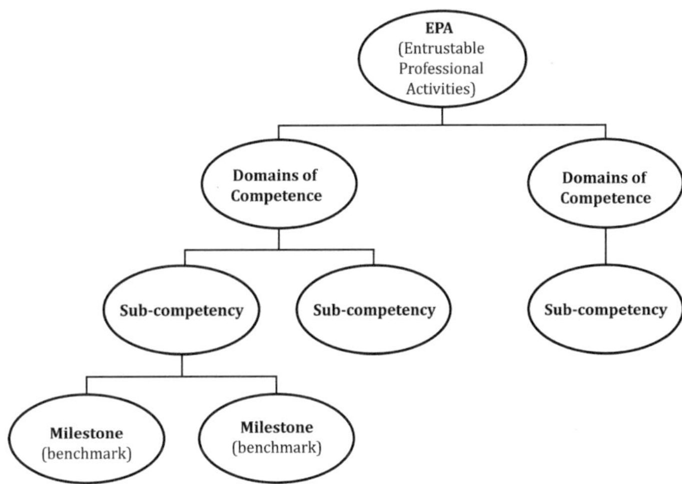

FIGURE 3.1 Depiction of EPAs, competencies, and milestones

In fact, the orthopaedic surgery milestones that have been developed have met with criticism. Van Heest and Dougherty (2015) argued that some procedural milestones may need to be modified to reflect more common procedures in orthopaedic surgery, and advocated for more research on appropriate assessment methods and tools. In addition, these authors argued that the milestones should undergo further research to establish them as valid metrics at the individual and program levels. Research must continue to establish strong and valid assessment tools for the milestones that are pertinent to surgical practice [12].

Backward Design: A Method for Writing Competency-Based Curriculum

Conducting a Needs Analysis

The first step in creating a competency-based curriculum is conducting a needs analysis to determine the key concepts and skills that are taught on a specific rotation or educational experience. A needs analysis should incorporate accreditation requirements, current gaps in the curriculum, and best educational practices in the specialty. A needs analysis will determine where a particular rotation or educational experience curriculum may need to be revised. Some programs may have an educational committee that can be charged to do this work. Other programs may need to create one and should include the program director, core clinical faculty from different subspecialties, and residents. Newer program directors may need to consult with or survey their subspecialty peers at the institution. Consulting with program directors from other institutions may also be helpful.

Writing competency-based curriculum for other educational experiences in the program is strongly suggested. These educational experiences may include didactics, simulation, journal clubs, quality improvement curriculum, etc. Using a standardized process, such as the one described, may be helpful. Utilizing the help of others, such as the Educational Committee within the program, key clinical faculty, senior residents or fellows, and program coordinators, may reduce the burden on the program director.

It is important to refer to the ACGME accreditation requirements in order to ensure that the curriculum meets appropriate standards, and to remain aware of ACGME updates to these standards. The ACGME Common Program requirements are a set of requirements common to all training programs, regardless of specialty. These requirements can be found on the ACGME website [13]. The specific curricular requirements for Orthopaedic Surgery Residency and Orthopaedic Surgery Fellowships are found on the ACGME website [14]. Program requirements are categorized as core, outcome, or detail. Core requirements refer to essential educational structures, processes, or resources required across all graduate training programs. Outcome requirements refer to measureable educational outcomes characterized as the knowledge, skills, or attitudes residents or fellows should demonstrate at key points in training. Detail requirements describe specific structures, processes, or resources required to meet the core requirements.

Other important sources to review include:

1. A review of the orthopaedic surgery milestones [11].
2. Current curriculum for each rotation.
3. A focused discussion, with residents and core clinical faculty, to determine whether there are content gaps, procedural gaps, or opportunities for improvement in the current curriculum: Information gleaned from the ACGME annual review process may also help to identify curricular gaps.
4. Feedback from Clinical Learning Environment Review (CLER) visits can be useful.
5. A discussion with the Designated Institutional Official (DIO) to determine if there is a plan to develop institutional curricula, with a surgical focus, for the four competencies: Interpersonal and Communication Skills, Professionalism, Practice-based Learning and Improvement, and Systems-based Practice.
6. A review of board certification requirements.
7. Curricula from other institutions.

Writing competency-based curricula for an orthopaedic surgery residency is a time-consuming task, but can be made easier by using an instructional design model to align outcomes (milestones) with objectives and competencies. Backward design is a three-step goal-directed process to align outcomes and curriculum with national standards [15]. Backward design is predicated on the following principle identified by Stephen Covey: "Begin with the end in mind" [16]. It is important to know the end result (educational outcome) and to construct curriculum to meet that result. In medical education, curriculum is generally constructed beginning with content and, then, attempting to link content to outcomes. This method often falls short in identifying specific outcomes, and communicating those outcomes to learners. The backward design model consists of three steps: identify desired results (outcomes such as milestones), determine acceptable evidence (assessment methods or tools), and plan learning experiences and instruction (objectives and teaching strategies). Backward design encourages an educational focus on the outcomes of a particular educational experience, and is an instructional design model directly in alignment with competency-based education. Figure 3.2 describes a step-by-step guide that can be used by program directors and faculty to create competency-based curriculum.

This guide contains components of backward design principles, which have been blended with ACGME accreditation requirements, providing a systematic process for creating curriculum. Program directors should begin by including a broad description of what the resident or fellow might learn during this rotation. The purpose of this description is to help orient the learner to the overall structure of the rotation. It may also be helpful to include an overall description of the setting, any specific requirements, level of supervision, any educational resources provided, and any other important features of this rotation. Once the description is written, the step-by-step guide can be useful in articulating the goals and objectives and educational outcomes of the rotation or educational experience.

Milestones (Identify Desired Results)

Resident performance on the ACGME Orthopaedic Surgery Milestones is the educational outcome expected at the end of each rotation. The milestones may vary from rotation to rotation, and not all milestones or competencies may be addressed on a particular rotation or educational experience. Program directors should list the specific milestones (outcomes) that are covered by the rotation in their curriculum document. Many orthopaedic surgery rotations may last a few months, and occur multiple times during training. The curricular document should list each iteration (PGY2, 3, etc.) and reflect the milestones for that particular iteration. The milestones described for the rotation may remain fairly consistent over the training period; however, resident or fellow progress on the milestones should increase as they become competent or proficient. Specifying the

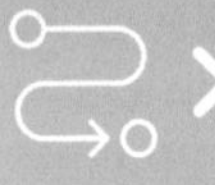

DESCRIPTION OF ROTATION

-Write a broad description of the rotation including what the resident might learn, overall description of setting, any specific requirements, educational resources, etc.

1

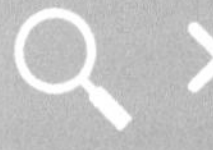

MILESTONES ADDRESSED ON THIS ROTATION

-Milestones are the educational outcomes of the rotation.
-List the milestones that are covered by the rotation in the curriculum document. If residents rotate more than once during their residency, list the milestones for each iteration by year.

2

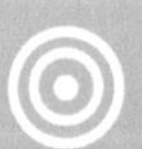

IDENTIFY EVIDENCE: ASSESSMENT METHODS

-List assessment methods or tools that will be used to assess residents.
-Consider using an assessment system that contains methods such as: direct observation, multisource feedback, and performance audit.

3

ROTATION GOALS

-List rotational goals.
-Goals are broad overarching statements of what a resident should learn.

4

ROTATION OBJECTIVES

- Objectives describe specific knowledge, skills or attitudes.
     -Link the objective to milestone(s).

5

Not all competencies or sub-competencies may be covered during a specific rotation

FIGURE 3.2 A step-by-step guide to create competency-based curriculum

milestones and level of performance to be reached by trainees helps them develop a road map for learning.

Assessment Methods or Tools (Identify Evidence)

This second step in the backward design model articulates appropriate assessment methods or tools to provide evidence for attainment of the milestones covered on the rotation and link the methods or tool to the milestones. The linking can be done by using codes or abbreviations. Multiple assessment tools, reflective of an overall assessment system, should be used, and aggregated to form a snapshot of resident or fellow performance on particular milestones. Important assessment methods to consider include longitudinal direct observation tools, multisource feedback, and performance audits. These assessment methods capture a picture of a resident's actual performance. Additional assessment tools might include case logs, in-training examination scores, patient surveys, simulation, and rating scales. The rotation curriculum should list the specific assessment methods or tools so trainees can identify how they will be assessed and the certifying body can see the process for evaluation. The ACGME Milestones Guidebook provides an overview of milestones, assessment, and best practices related to creating an assessment system [17]. Assessment tools should be specified for each time residents or fellows rotate through a particular rotation. It may also be helpful to include statements about when and how feedback occurs. Helping residents incorporate feedback into their own learning plan helps them to refine knowledge and skills.

Plan Learning Experiences

Rotation Goals

Educational goals are broad statements describing what the learner will gain from the rotation or educational experience. Goals are not necessarily measurable and, typically, provide the "big picture" of the rotation or educational experience. Goals for a rotation do not contain discrete knowledge, skills, or attitudes which can be measured. Goals articulate the overarching concepts trainees will learn during the experience throughout all iterations of the rotation and at the same time should address the six competency domains. In some ways, they might be thought of as a "mission statement" for the rotation.

Examples

1. On the ortho trauma rotations, residents will learn to provide culturally competent patient-centered care to trauma patients, and communicate effectively with the patient's families, and the care team.
2. On the ortho trauma rotations, residents will self-reflect to identify their own limitations, develop a plan to remediate those learning gaps, and use evidence-based approach to care.

Objectives

Objectives, on the other hand, are statements that reflect the knowledge, skills, or attitudes residents should acquire during the rotation. Knowledge objectives reflect the concrete knowledge trainees will gain on a rotation as a result of various educational experiences, and are generally acquired through didactics, self-directed learning, or feedback. Skill objectives reflect a wide variety of skill sets such as procedural skill sets, communication skill sets, diagnostic and patient management skill sets, among many others. Attitude objectives represent those attitudes that trainees develop as part of the process of professional identity formation.

Writing objectives can be challenging and poses a number of questions which may require consultation with peers in and out of the home institution. How does one choose the core concepts taught on the rotation? How granular does one get when writing objectives? How does one identify key concepts taught on a rotation in an efficient manner, given the complexity of medical training? How does one link these objectives to the competencies and milestones?

For many orthopaedic surgery programs, rotations on a particular service (i.e., orthopaedic trauma) may occur multiple times throughout training due to staffing requirements and availability and level of training material. It is important to start by delineating core concepts residents will learn during the rotation, and to group objectives based on the year of training. Given the complexity of medical training, rotation objectives should specify the broad skills and knowledge obtained on the rotation, without becoming too granular. For rotations that span years, it is helpful to separate out the objectives by year so trainees and faculty can identify skill sets and expectations for learning and assessment. The art is to specify the objectives for each year without being too restrictive or overly vague in order to facilitate implementation and assessment.

Rotation objectives should be structured to provide an action verb that reflects application of knowledge and demonstration of skill. Bloom's Taxonomy is a well-recognized resource for identifying appropriate verbs that reflect increasing knowledge and skills [18]. Verbs such as demonstrate, appraise, maintain, practice, or perform are examples of verbs that require more complex cognitive skills. Verbs, such as "know" or "understand," may not communicate to trainees and faculty the complexity of the skill or knowledge required in a residency or fellowship setting. A simple format, such as the one that follows, may be helpful:

> At the end of the rotation, the (insert year of residency or fellowship) should (insert verb) (insert skill). (Code for milestone(s)).

Link the objective to the particular milestone by using abbreviations in parenthesis. By linking the objective to a specific milestone, it will guide the program director in identifying the particular milestone(s) to be assessed on the rotation. See Fig. 3.3 for an overview of this process.

Some rotations in orthopaedic surgery are repeated numerous times throughout training. The expectations of the residents and their ability to perform tasks increase with each iteration of the rotation. It is important to capture the increased complexity

Description of Rotation
- Include an overall description including setting, level of supervision, any educational resources provided, and any other important features of this rotation.

Identify Desired Results: Milestones Addressed on this Rotation:
- List which milestones are addressed on this rotation

Identify Evidence: Assessment Methods:
- List assessment tools used on this rotation.

Rotation Goals:
- List broad educational goals for the rotation.

Rotation Objectives
- Identify key concepts residents learn on the rotation
- Determine which action verbs accurately depict skill level
- Link these objectives with the specific milestones
- If residents are assigned multiple times to this rotation during training, then separate out the objectives by years (i.e. PGY1, PGY2, PGY3, PGY4, PGY5). The objectives should reflect increases in skill or knowledge and an increase in independence.
- Not all competencies or sub-competencies may be covered during a specific rotation.

FIGURE 3.3 Overview of the curriculum design process

in the objectives. One way to do this is to use verbs that reflect increasing levels of complexity or skills. The following objectives illustrate examples of the increased complexity of skills reflected in the objectives for an orthopaedic trauma rotation. Pay close attention to the knowledge and skills required for a rotation and capture those in the objectives.

PGY 2 years (length of time is 3 months)

1. The resident will demonstrate basics of adult trauma inpatient management (MK, PC).
2. The resident will demonstrate basic surgical skills by assisting in the OR and perform simple cases (i.e., fixation of a fracture) under supervision (MK, PC).
3. The resident will demonstrate the ability to manage straightforward postsurgical cases (MK, PC).

PGY 4

1. The resident will be able to interpret advanced imaging studies for various orthopaedic conditions (MK, PC).
2. The resident will be able to perform simple fixation of fractures of ankle, hip, etc. (MK, PC).
3. The resident will perform effective clinical assessments in the orthopaedic surgery clinic (MK, PC).

PGY 5

1. The resident will perform appropriate surgical procedures on a full range of fractures or dislocations of moderate complexity (MK, PC).
2. The resident will perform complete and effective assessment in clinic on a wide range of complex patients (MK, PC).
3. The resident will supervise junior residents and other members of the health care team in the examination of the patient and development of a treatment plan (MK, PC, ICS).

Rotations which only occur once during training, such as pediatric orthopaedics, may only need one set of objectives covering the six domains of competence.

Putting It All Together

Competency-based curriculum is challenging to write and it is critical that the outcomes, assessment methods, and teaching objectives and strategies be carefully aligned. It may be helpful to assemble a team of key clinical faculty who are familiar with each of the rotations and begin to identify where milestones are taught, the assessment system and where specific tools fit in, as well as key objectives for rotations. A tip to writing objectives is to identify the key concepts or skills that residents need to acquire during that rotation. Once those key concepts are identified, using the format described above may help with writing the objective. The objectives should link to a milestone(s), and clearly displaying that link by the method described above will help the faculty and resident know what they need to teach/learn, and specifically what milestone is addressed.

Challenges

Writing a competency-based curriculum may feel a lot like "rearranging the deck chairs," but it is necessary to provide a road map for trainees and faculty that clearly lays out learning expectations, assessment methods, and milestones for achievement. Creating this type of curriculum requires time, a precious resource in graduate medical education. Hopefully, the step-by-step guide will minimize faculty time by providing a systematic process to create competency-based curriculum. In some cases, the current curriculum can be transformed into a competency-based curriculum with minimal effort.

It is critical to keep in mind that EPAs may come to orthopaedic surgery. EPAs, which are broad professional skill sets measured primarily by direct observation or other workplace assessment, are composed of a number of competency domains and will add another layer of complexity to the curriculum. Ideally, they can be incorporated into this template at the beginning by simply adding a separate heading and linking competencies and milestones to them. Conversations about developing standardized curriculum in orthopaedic surgery at the national level may help program directors organize and implement competency-based education more easily.

Conclusion

Clear, concise objectives linked to assessment methods and milestones will create a common understanding of the content of the rotation for the faculty and the resident. Backward design is an instructional design model that provides clarity in highlighting educational outcomes, identifying assessment methods, and linking those to the actual content of the rotation [15]. Following the stepwise process described in this chapter helps faculty create rotation-specific curricula that link educational outcomes with teaching content.

References

1. Batalden P, Leach D, Swing S, Dreyfus H, Dreyfus S. General competencies and accreditation in graduate medical education. Health Aff (Millwood). 21(5):103–11.

 2. Swing SR. The ACGME outcome project: retrospective and prospective. Med Teach. 2007 Sep;29(7):648–54.
 3. Frank JR, Mungroo R, Ahmad Y, Wang M, De Rossi S, Horsley T. Toward a definition of competency-based education in medicine: a systematic review of published definitions. Med Teach. 2010;32(8):631–7.
 4. Frank JR, Snell LS, Cate OT, Holmboe ES, Carraccio C, Swing SR, et al. Competency-based medical education: theory to practice. Med Teach. 2010;32(8):638–45.
 5. Carraccio CL, Englander R. From Flexner to competencies. Acad Med. 2013;88(8):1067–73.
 6. Nasca TJ, Philibert I, Brigham T, Flynn TC. The next GME accreditation system—rationale and benefits. N Engl J Med. 2012;366(11):1051–6.
 7. Dreyfus SE. The five-stage model of adult skill acquisition. Bull Sci Technol Soc. 2004;24(3):177–81.
 8. Carraccio C, Englander R, Gilhooly J, Mink R, Hofkosh D, Barone MA, et al. Building a framework of Entrustable professional activities, supported by competencies and milestones, to bridge the educational continuum. Acad Med. 2016;92(3):324–30.
 9. Caverzagie KJ, Cooney TG, Hemmer PA, Berkowitz L. The development of Entrustable professional activities for internal medicine residency training. Acad Med. 2015;90(4):479–84.
10. ten Cate O, Scheele F. Competency-based postgraduate training: can we bridge the gap between theory and clinical practice? Acad Med. 2007;82(6):542–7.
11. Stern PJ, Albanese S, Bostrom M, Day CS, Frick SL, Hopkinson W, et al. Orthopaedic surgery milestones. J Grad Med Educ. 2013;5(1 Suppl 1):36–58.
12. Van Heest AE, Dougherty PJ. CORR® curriculum—orthopaedic education: operative assessment and the ACGME milestones: time for change. Clin Orthop Relat Res. 2015;473(3):775–8.
13. ACGME Common Program Requirements [Internet]. [cited 2016 Oct 18]. https://www.acgme.org/Portals/0/PFAssets/ProgramRequirements/CPRs_07012016.pdf
14. ACGME Program Requirements for Graduate Medical Education in Orthopaedic Surgery [Internet]. [cited 2016 Oct 18] http://www.acgme.org/Portals/0/PFAssets/ProgramRequirements/260_orthopaedic_surgery_2016.pdf
15. Wiggins GP, McTighe J. Understanding by design. 2nd ed. Alexandria, VA: Association for Supervision and Curriculum Development; 2005.

16. Covey SR. The seven habits of highly effective people: restoring the character ethic. New York: Fireside Books; 1989.
17. Holmboe ES, Edgar L, Hamstra S. The milestones guidebook [Internet]. [cited 2016 Dec 6]. http://www.acgme.org/Portals/0/MilestonesGuidebook.pdf
18. Bloom B. Bloom's taxonomy action verbs [Internet]. [cited 2016 Dec 8]. http://www.fresnostate.edu/academics/oie/documents/assesments/Blooms Level.pdf.

Chapter 4
Teaching as Coaching

Deana M. Mercer, Marlene A. DeMaio, Daniel C. Wascher, Paul G. Echols, and Robert C. Schenck Jr.

Relevance and Benefits of Coaching: From Residency to Practice

Coaching is considered a learned skill. There are those who are innately better at the challenge, but coaching is an ability that is learned, and even those successful "natural" coaches can improve their abilities. A basic understanding of the different components involved in the process can be helpful in guiding the coach, which in turn creates a platform for the "coached" to be successful. Coaching is an accepted practice in many professions and activities, particularly sports, performing arts, music, and public speaking. Numerous textbooks and popular instructional books describe and tout the irreplaceable benefits of good coaching. It has not been traditionally embraced by surgeons, most likely because the

D.M. Mercer, MD (✉) • D.C. Wascher, MD
P.G. Echols, MD • R.C. Schenck Jr., MD
Department of Orthopaedics and Rehabilitation,
The University of New Mexico Health Sciences Center,
Albuquerque, NM 87131-0001, USA
e-mail: dmercer@salud.unm.edu

M.A. DeMaio, MD
Department of Orthopaedic Surgery, Perelman School of Medicine,
University of Pennsylvania, Philadelphia, PA, USA

© Springer International Publishing AG 2018
P.J. Dougherty, B.L. Joyce (eds.), *The Orthopedic Educator*,
DOI 10.1007/978-3-319-62944-5_4

majority of teaching uses the instructor/teacher-centered and apprenticeship methods. However, coaching has particular relevance and benefits for anyone learning orthopaedics. In this chapter, we present benefits of, examples of, and general guidelines for coaching.

Coaching is important in that orthopaedic surgeons in the modern healthcare environment cannot learn everything needed for a successful 30-year career from lectures, printed materials (books, journals), videos, residency, or fellowship. Many challenges that physicians will encounter in their career are poorly taught during training and are rarely the subject of presentations at meetings or journal articles. Some examples of these challenges are acquiring leadership skills, navigating changes in practice, managing an orthopaedic business, or developing research ideas. Atul Gawande was one of the early proponents of "being coached" as a surgeon in a similar successful approach he had used in playing tennis [1]. In the end, nothing really beats experience, and learning from the experienced is invaluable be it sports, medicine, or even parenting. Coaches are those that have had years of opportunity to make mistakes and learned valuable lessons from those errors. This knowledge from experience can be transferred to the learner in many ways, one of them being one-on-one coaching. The advantage of one-on-one coaching is that it is individualized and focused on the needs of the student. Each learner has different needs; the coach is responsible for identifying these needs and recognizing the best method of instruction for that particular person. Lastly, coaching involves observing, with recommendations for the coached to practice or incorporate suggestions in their daily work … or tennis.

Most commonly, the most successful coaches are those who have had years of opportunity to garner and reflect on experience, which includes wins and losses, successes and failures, as well as perfection and mistakes. Lauded coaches commonly have the ability to understand outcomes, causal relationships, and preparation. Such individuals are able to see why what seemed like a good idea was not. They are able to backpedal and see where the unintended consequences occurred and then make adjustments. Interestingly, some of the best coaches were average or below-average performers in their areas of expertise.

Coaching and Mentoring: There Is a Difference

There are differences between coaches and mentors. Interestingly, a coach may have skills that include mentoring but a mentor is not a coach (Table 4.1). Both may be focused on accomplishing a task, but the manner of the approach is different.

Coach: The word "coach" stems from the Hungarian word *kocsi*, meaning to transport people from where they are to where they want to be [2]. In today's world, a coach is usually defined as someone who teaches and trains an athlete or a performer. It is a private instructor who has expertise in a particular subject. The first known use of the word "coach" as an instructor or teacher dates back to 1830 at Oxford, when the coach would "carry" the student through the examination [3]. In sports, the first known use of the word was in Europe in the 1860s, in which the word was used to describe the instructor of the 1859 English Cricket Team [3, 4]. Today, almost all professional athletes and performers have at least one coach. A modern coach may be a teacher, leader, motivator, and critic. However, the use of coaches is rare within medical professions [5].

TABLE 4.1 Coach[a] versus mentor

Variable	Mentor	Coach[a]
Age	Often older than student	Any age
Life skills	Yes	Often no
Knowledge and education	Yes	No
Team skills	No	Yes
Task	Yes	Yes
Involved in a sport	Often no	Yes

[a]Coaches can be mentors: fairness, integrity, motivation

Mentor: Similar to a coach, a mentor is someone who teaches, helps, or advises a less experienced, often younger individual. A mentor is a trusted counselor and guide, who can also be a tutor but most importantly is a role model. Learners tend to hold their mentors in high regard and attempt to emulate their skills and persona. This concept of mentorship stems back to ancient Greece [6]. Mentor was the son of Heracles and also a friend of Odysseus, and Odysseus entrusted Mentor with the education of his son Telemachus. The first modern known usage of "mentor" was in 1699 in *Les Aventures de Télémaque* by François Fénelon [7]. Mentor was the main character in this book that remained popular until the eighteenth century. Mentor denounced war and imperialism while promoting a federation of nations to work together, and altruism. The character enforced the continued use of the noun mentor who wisely advised and taught.

Although mentors and coaches both aim to assist learners, the method of guidance is different. Simply put, mentors are role models, whereas coaches are critics. Other distinctions include long-term or short-term instruction and general or specific goals, respectively [8]. The coach aims to help address immediate problems for the learner, with the goal being improvement of a particular performance feature.

So What Is a Coach?

A coach is a teacher, leader, motivator, and critic, with typically more experience than the learner. Interestingly coaches may not be the most talented performers in their field but compensate for lack of skill with a tireless study of the "game." The coach helps the athlete/surgeon capitalize on individual strengths and helps the player/surgeon adjust for deficits. The coach typically stays in the background, observes, teaches strategy and technique, and also organizes a team to maximize overall performance (Table 4.2).

In a coaching relationship, both the coach and the athlete are invested. Chemistry does matter, and thus some coach-athlete relationships do not work and this is an important note for the

TABLE 4.2 Surgical techniques

Technique	Definition[a]
Competency	An ability or skill
Proficiency	Advancement in knowledge or skill; the quality or state of being proficient
Mastery	Knowledge or skill that makes one master of a subject; command

[a]Merriam Webster Dictionary. Competency, proficiency, mastery (2017). https://www.merriam-webster.com/. Accessed 10 Jan 2017 [9]

surgeon looking for a coach. The sooner this chemistry is apparent, the better, as both parties can then move forward or reevaluate the relationship. With coaching, both parties share ideas and can benefit and learn from each other. Criticism is always difficult to accept, yet learners, when employing the coaching model, must accept scrutiny to allow the coach to identify not only magnificence but also deficiencies. Similar to chemistry, the sooner this exchange of information is streamlined, the sooner can coaching-type relationships become effective and productive. For surgeons with an independent mind set and confidence, the importance of accepting scrutiny and criticism is a necessary ingredient for success. If the surgeon is not "coachable" then the concept and approach of coaching are not going to be successful. From the start, a coach must express what the learner does not want to see or hear to help maximize performance. Good coaches break performance down into components and critique and enforce deliberate practice. Obstacles to being a good coach include a lack of attention to detail, rigidity, and ego. Clearly the successful coach, especially in medicine, must be facile in communicating, especially with topics that the coached may not want to hear.

Coaching in Teaching

Coaching is directly related to the teacher quality. In general, younger teachers are more amenable. Obstacles to being a good coach include fear, unhealthy paranoia, ego, and insecurities. Good coaches break performance down into components and critique and enforce deliberate practice [1].

Coaching in Surgery

As noted above, Atul Gawande popularized the concept of coaching in surgery with his essay in the *New Yorker* [1]. He noted that after 8 years of practice, his skills and complication rate had plateaued. He wanted to continue to improve as a surgeon but found an absence of relevant mentors or coaches. Gawande noted that traditionally, once a surgeon completed residency and fellowship training, no formal method existed for improving one's skills under the guidance of a "coach." He found personalized and individualized instruction lacking. He approached a senior surgeon to specifically review his performance and from this improved multiple parts of the procedure.

Gwande cites Jim Knight, Ph.D., Director of the Kansas Coaching Project, to emphasize some key elements that he concluded were important for surgical coaching. These points are as follows: learning may be directly related to the quality of the teacher; coached teachers are more effective than teachers who are not coached; younger teachers are more amenable to being coached; and some concerns that the teachers had about being coached included fear and insecurity.

Furthermore, in surgery, coaching may be seen as a sign of weakness and inadequacy. There is a perception that only incompetent surgeons need coaches. Yet, we know that virtually all successful professional athletes, singers, and Oscar-winning actors have coaches throughout their career, even when at the "top of their game." Among athletes and performers, society recognizes the difficulty of working without a coach in realizing potential—and the subsequent risk of becoming stagnant. This concept has great value for the medical/surgical world.

Sachdeva et al. further commented that in the world of surgery, having a coach is often perceived as lacking skill, not as an effort toward improving outcomes and efficiency [10].

In Orthopaedics, at The University of New Mexico, the concept of coaching is welcomed and has been accepted and promulgated by senior surgeons and the chair (Fig. 4.1) [11]. Clearly, patients may be suspicious of the concept of the coached surgeon, believing that surgeons who need coaching may not be the most qualified to perform treatment. Additionally, surgical colleagues may also see the presence of a coach as a sign of faltering confidence. This negative connotation of coaching in surgery may stem from the practice of mandated proctoring of young surgeons or those with unacceptable complication rates. It is important to differentiate between the voluntary request for a coach to maximize potential and forced observation of a coach to ensure patient safety (Table 4.3).

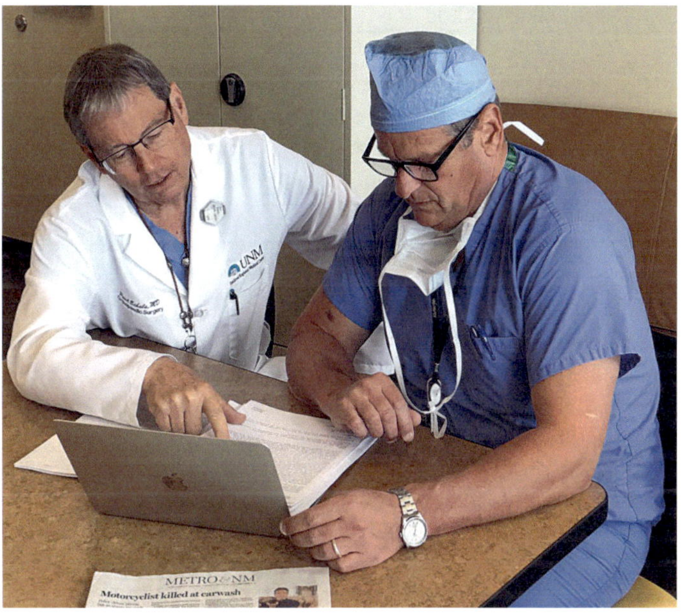

FIGURE 4.1 Coaching requires introducing the coach and obtaining permission from the patient. We routinely request permission in clinic during our standard preoperative visit and then introduce the patient the day of surgery

TABLE 4.3 Tasks for the surgical coach and the surgeon being coached

Tasks of surgical coach	Tasks of surgeon being coached
Areas to evaluate	Define the area(s) of interest
Specific task	Be open to discussion and improving
Surgical technique	Develop a plan to continue improvement
Efficiency	
Communication	
Determine general concepts	
Identify areas for improvement	
Optimal teaching method	

Coaching takes time. However, as Oliver Cromwell said, "He who stops being better stops being good" [12]. Practice demands (outcomes, leadership, business, and government mandates) are ever increasing; it is difficult to take the time to meet with coaches, hear their criticism, and work to overcome weaknesses. The relationship between the coach and the coached individual must be developed, and an understanding of the goals and methods of communication must be clear. It may take time to iron out the details of the coaching relationship, and it may take several iterations before the approach becomes clear. But in our experience and that of others, coaching is an integral part of improving our abilities, stretching our success to new goals.

In today's world, the crowd is watching. Government and insurance companies are tracking our outcomes as physicians and adjusting payment accordingly. Healthcare systems routinely survey customers regarding provider performance. Our patients are rating us, and potential patients are using those ratings to select us. Improving knowledge of care and refining our skills are necessary and beneficial for both surgeons and patients. Coaching, when employed with understanding, humility, and "coachability," is an ideal avenue for success.

Coaching in Orthopaedics

In orthopaedics, little formal implementation exists regarding the concept of coaching. Coaching is not actively promoted by accreditation boards (e.g., Accreditation Council for Graduate Medical Education, Association of American Medical Colleges, American Academy of Orthopaedic Surgeons, or American Board of Orthopaedic Surgeons) or applied in surgical practice. Conceptually, it could be a powerful tool in residency when acquiring knowledge and learning skills is the key. Although the concept of lifelong learning is encouraged from medical school onward, coaching is not a traditional part of professional development. As part of obtaining and maintaining certification, coaching could also have a powerful role. There is certainly more to the practice of orthopaedic surgery than continuing medical education and score and record examinations, which have their place in the objective monitoring of lifelong learning. The American Board of Orthopaedic Surgery requires a program to maintain board certification, yet this is primarily based on self-study and attendance of medical-education conferences [13]. These traditional forms of orthopaedic education have an important role but may lack the individualized critical feedback and suggestions for improvement, which a coach provides. The use of a coach can have great potential for helping orthopaedists stay on top of their game. Additionally, a surgeon may wish to resume a procedure that was once part of his or her practice in the past and identifies the need to improve.

We must also recognize that, in addition to the reluctance of surgeons to be coached, there is also a shortage of coaches in orthopaedics. National leadership and surgical organizations should be encouraged to initiate a program to train orthopaedic coaches, with some examples having been attempted in the past with limited success. This coaching education would allow experienced physicians—whose "playing days" can be improved by becoming a player coach so to speak—to remain actively engaged in promoting surgical excellence. The results of such collaboration would benefit not only the coach and the learner, but most importantly our patients (Fig. 4.2).

There have been several formal discussions of coaching in orthopaedics. Two were part of national orthopaedic meetings and one is a chapter in a book authored by a specialty-trained orthopaedic surgeon. Interestingly, all of these presentations involve surgeons in the subspecialty of sports medicine, most likely stemming from the observed benefits of sports coaching.

During the annual meeting of the American Orthopaedic Society of Sports Medicine in 2013, there was a symposium on coaching [14]. The observations and recommendations were presented for two surgeons who were coached by a more senior surgeon. One scenario was in the operating room and the other was in the clinic. Another symposium was dedicated to this topic at the 2014 Combined AOA for the USA and Canada [11] (Table 4.4). The definitions, applications, and benefits of coaching were reviewed. A structured example of

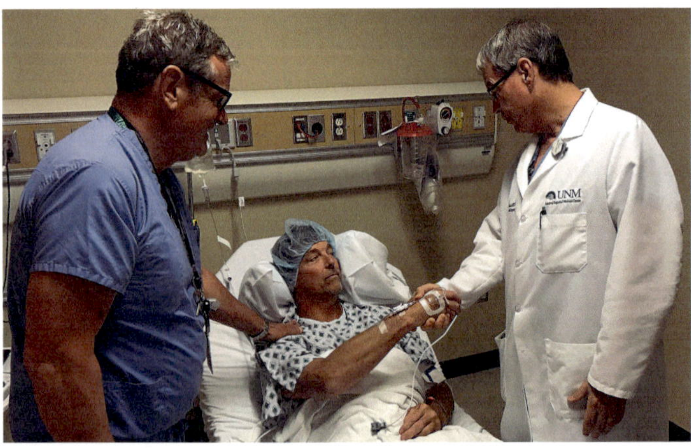

FIGURE 4.2 Coach observes and takes notes for the operating-room day from start to finish. Strategies for timesaving and intraoperative decision making are many things that are coachable

Table 4.4   Coaching concepts from sports applicable to surgical coaching[a]

Name of coach	Coach's goal	Quote
Scotty Bowman	Brings out the greatness in players	"If you are going to win games, you had better be ready to adapt"
Herb Brooks	Understands the need for the coach	"You don't have enough talent to win on talent alone"
Sean Foley	Can avoid the limelight. The emphasis on student	"I'm the help, not the talent"
Kelly Amonte Hiller	Directs improvement	"The right coach transports you from where you are to where you want to be"
Phil Jackson	Understands his or her own strengths. Some of the best coaches were not exceptional athletes	"Wisdom is always an overmatch for strength"
Mike Krzyzewski	Leads	"I don't look at myself as a basketball coach, I look at myself as a leader who happens to coach basketball"
Tom Landry	Critic: Improves *you*	"A coach is someone who tells you what you don't want to hear, who has you see what you don't want to see, so you can be who you have always known you could be"
Vince Lombardi	Motivator: Offers encouragement, pushes to excel	"Perfection is not attainable, but if we chase perfection, we can catch excellence"
Joe Paterno	Improves current skills	"In coaching, we have to get to the soul of the people we are dealing with"

(continued)

TABLE 4.4 (continued)

Name of coach	Coach's goal	Quote
Pat Summit	Teaches new skills	"Change is risky. It is not as risky, however, as standing still"
John Wooden	Coach as critic: Points out mistakes; corrects flaws	"If you don't have time to do it right, when will you have time to do it over?"
		"It's what you learn after you know it all that counts."

[a]Adapted from DeMaio M, Schenck R, Wascher D, Miller M. Coaching in orthopaedic surgery. Presented at: The Combined Meeting of the AOA and the COA 2014, June 18–21, 2014, Montreal, Canada [11]

a formal coach (author PE) working with an accomplished surgeon (author RS) resuming total knee arthroplasty in 2013 was presented. A quality analysis of the first 30 cases was part of the report to the surgeon's Credentials Committee. The first 100 cases were followed for a minimum of 2 years. The importance of "chemistry" between the coach and the surgeon was emphasized. The lessons learned from this experience were that coaches may formally advise to improve technique and that both surgeons benefited from the experience. Benefits are many and include the opportunity to build a relationship, and provide great satisfaction for a senior surgeon functioning as a coach and giving back information. The coached surgeon has the opportunity to learn in ways that are unique and differ significantly from standard continuing medical education that is hands on and immediate. A subtle but important benefit is that, once having gone through the process, the coached surgeon has a new understanding that can be suggested or offered to others in need of improved behaviors or techniques, through a very unique learning process.

The Coach

Christopher S. Ahmad, M.D., authored *Skill: 40 Principles that Surgeons, Athletes, and other Elite Performers Use to Achieve Mastery* [15]. Chapter 37 is devoted to coaching as is Reflections 5. He points out several very important observations as seen in Table 4.5. Importantly, he recommends teaching. He states: "Coach with excellence to achieve your personal pursuit of greatness. Every person you coach is a mirror for you." Further, he cites Daniel Coyle's *The Little Book of Talent* to provide some guidelines for coaches (Table 4.6).

The age-old adage, "when the student is ready, the teacher will appear," is a long-held understanding in the world of learning. But the balance of student readiness and finding the right coach can take time, some effort, and several trials before the match is right. The student must be ready to

TABLE 4.5 Major points to improve skill by coaching as described by Christopher S. Ahmad[a]

Major points in coaching
Take prolific notes, often
Distinguish between hard and soft skills
Obsess over details, dissect
Review and evaluate observations, experiences
Perform mental practice, practice, and review
Learn from the masters
Incorporate "lessons learned" from mistakes
Keep a broad view and an open mind
Teach

[a]Adapted from Ahmad CS (2015) Chapter 37. Be a better coach. pp. 128–133 and Additional Reflections, Reflection 5. Coaching pp. 165–171. In: Skill. Lead Player LLC, Brooklyn, NY [15]

TABLE 4.6 Rules for coaches as described by Christopher S. Ahmad after Daniel Coyle in *The Little Book of Talent*[a]

Number	Rule
1	Use the first few seconds to connect on an emotional level
2	Avoid giving long speeches; instead deliver vivid chunks of information
3	Be allergic to mushy language
4	Make a scorecard for your students
5	Broaden view to connect with the coached learner
6	Aim to create independent learners

[a]Adapted from Ahmad CS (2015) Be a better coach. In: Skill. Lead Player LLC, Brooklyn, NY, pp. 128–133 [15]

accept criticism and guidance without being defensive, whereas the coach must be able to connect with the student on an emotional level. Chemistry is vital to the success of the endeavor. Furthermore, coaches should avoid long speeches and instead deliver succinct information in a factual manner, which is pertinent to the situation and topic. Embellishment and exaggeration should be avoided. In addition to improving students' performance, an additional goal should be to help learners develop skills to become a coach for future surgeons [1].

We can all do better as orthopaedic caretakers, researchers, leaders, and educators. While concepts and technology change, our knowledge and skills in all areas tend to plateau. Coaching is a method to improve one's performance. Becoming comfortable with being coached may take some time, preparation, and self-awareness. Embracing this concept can be difficult for a surgeon, as one's deficiencies must be acknowledged. However, the insight and humility to utilize a coach can result in improved performance, increased confidence, and more successful patient outcomes (Fig. 4.3).

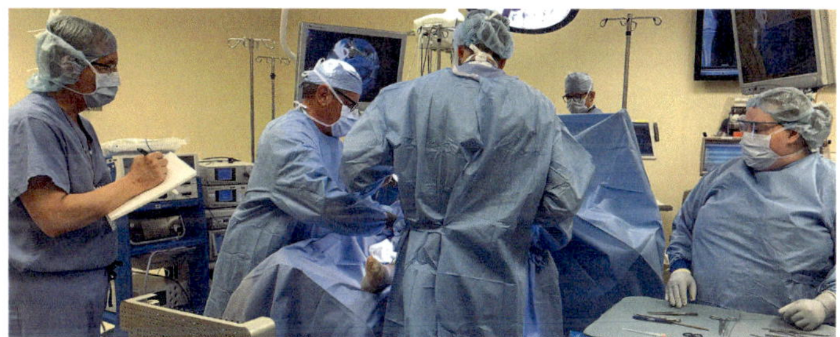

FIGURE 4.3 Coach and coached meet at the end of the day to discuss observations, ask questions, make recommendations, and plan for modifications in work or behavior

References

1. Gawande A. Personal best: top athletes and singers have coaches—should you? 2011. .The New Yorker 2011 issue. http://www.newyorker.com/magazine/2011/10/03/personal-best. Accessed 10 Jan 2017.
2. Pavlovic J, Stojnov D. Personal construct coaching. In: Winter DA, Reed N, editors. The Wiley handbook of personal construct psychology. Chichester: Wiley; 2016. p. 320–30.
3. Coach HD. In: Online Etymology Dictionary. 2017.http://www. etymonline.com/index.php?term=coach. Accessed 10 Jan 2017.
4. WL Murdoch. A chat about cricket. Longman's Magazine 1881;1:287–298.
5. Gifford GA, Fall LH. Doctor coach: A deliberate practice approach to teaching and learning clinical skills. Acad Med. 2014;89(2):272–6.
6. Mentor HD. In: Online Etymology Dictionary. 2017.http://www. etymonline.com/index.php?term=mentor. Accessed 10 Jan 2017.
7. Roberts A. The origins of the term mentor. Hist Educ Soc Bull. 1999;64:313–29.
8. Coaching and mentoring—the difference. 2015. Brefi Group Limited. http://www.brefigroup.co.uk/coaching/coaching_and_ mentoring.html. Accessed 10 Jan 2017.
9. Merriam Webster Dictionary. Competency, proficiency, mastery. 2017. https://www.merriam-webster.com/. Accessed 10 Jan 2017.

10. Sachdeva AK, Blair PG, Lupi LK. Education and training to address specific needs during the career progression of surgeons. Surg Clin N Am. 2016;96:115–28.
11. DeMaio M, Schenck R, Wascher D, Miller M. Coaching in orthopaedic surgery. Presented at: The Combined Meeting of the AOA and the COA 2014, June 18–21, 2014, Montreal, Canada.
12. He who stops being better stops being good. 2012. Burcu's Teaching and Learning Zone. http://btezcan.edublogs.org/2012/08/30/he-who-stops-being-better-stops-being-good-oliver-cromwell/. Accessed 10 Jan 2017.
13. Verify certification. Chapel Hill: The American Board of Orthopaedic Surgery. 2017. https://www.abos.org/verify-certification.aspx. Accessed 10 Jan 2017.
14. Gawande A, Taylor DC, Curl W, DeLee JC, Tolin BS. Improving your game: surgeons coaching surgeons. Symposium presented at AOSSM Annual Meeting 2013, July 11–14, Chicago.
15. Ahmad CS. Be a better coach. In: skill: 40 principles that surgeons, athletes, and other elite performers use to achieve mastery. Brooklyn: Lead Player, 2015. p. 128–33 and 165–71.

Chapter 5
Teaching Operative Skills

Paul J. Dougherty and A.E. Van Heest

Introduction

Medical education is experiential in nature. Medical students and residents learn through the experience of actually practicing medicine on patients, under the supervision of a fully trained physician. The resident surgeon must develop procedural skills so that a procedure can be done independently and competently upon graduation. Teaching operative skills is also experiential. Successful educators need to properly supervise residents, which is a skill that they will develop over time and with experience. New faculty are expected to educate residents, yet often are left to develop their own "operative teaching skill set" without any specific training or guidance. In the first 2 years of practice, a new faculty member is fresh out of fellowship, and needs to develop their own operative skills, yet at the same time is learning how to teach

P.J. Dougherty, MD (✉)
Department of Orthopaedic Surgery,
University of Florida College of Medicine—Jacksonville,
655 W 8th Street, 2nd Floor ACC, Jacksonville, FL 32209, USA
e-mail: paul.dougherty@jax.ufl.edu

A.E. Van Heest, MD
Department of Orthopaedic Surgery, University of Minnesota,
2450 Riverside Avenue South, Suite R200,
Minneapolis, MN 55454, USA

© Springer International Publishing AG 2018   77
P.J. Dougherty, B.L. Joyce (eds.), *The Orthopedic Educator*,
DOI 10.1007/978-3-319-62944-5_5

and supervise residents' operative skills, all while collecting cases for the American Board of Orthopaedic Surgery Part II examination! When starting out as a new faculty member, concerns about patient safety versus allowing the resident more hands-on experience tend to favor patient safety and, thus, provides less resident hands-on experience. This can lead to frustration for both faculty and residents. When comparing surgical residency programs to the nonsurgical programs, the major difference is the role of the faculty in teaching and supervising operative skills. This fundamental difference is grounded in the fact that motor skills, specifically the operative skills that allow for safe and consistent performance of a procedure, must be learned by deliberate practice.

Traditionally, surgical procedures have been taught through exposure to a large number of cases, augmented by self-directed reading and study. As a resident became more experienced, he or she was able to gain more autonomy in the operating room. See one, do one, teach one.

This paradigm no longer exists in surgical training. Several changes have occurred since 1999 in the structure of orthopaedic surgery (and graduate medical education) which have influenced the way we teach. Initially, the national restrictions of resident duty hours have limited resident exposure to large numbers of cases. Secondly, the Institute of Medicine has issued several warnings regarding the concerns of patient safety; this has increased the requirement for faculty to be directly present for surgical care of the patient. In most cases, faculty presence has decreased residents' autonomy in the operating room. The balance between education and safety of patients is a tension present in all graduate medical education programs, and is especially heightened during the performance of surgical procedures. Thirdly, the development by the ACGME of "general competencies" defined six areas considered important for the training of all doctors, not just orthopaedic surgeons. But a weakness was found with the six general competencies. Standards were not developed, much less assessment tools. The six general competencies include surgical procedures as a subset of patient care, and do not recognize the differences between teaching and assessing nonoperative patient care skills versus operative technical skills. Technical skills are a different skill set that needs separate teaching strategies and separate assessment tools. Often faculty were left wondering how competencies applied to what was being taught in orthopaedic surgery residency.

The purpose of this chapter is to provide a framework for teaching residents operative skills in the operating room or in a simulation center. A teaching framework can help faculty structure teaching in a way that promotes efficient use of teaching time and maximized resident learning.

Structured Teaching in the Operating Room

Roberts et al. [1] developed the BID model designed to provide a framework for faculty to follow during the teaching encounter to improve resident performance in an operative setting [1]. The BID model is described as briefing (B), intraoperative teaching (I), and debriefing (D). Preoperatively, a discussion or *briefing* (B) with the resident assesses the needs of this learner, and sets forth the performance improvement goals for the procedure. *Intraoperative teaching* (I) focuses on specific areas of performance related towards building on the skills of the individual learner. For example, a middle-level resident might focus on precise placement of a guide wire for an intramedullary nail. This technique is meant to guide a focused conversation to develop operative skill building and identify particular areas for improvement of the learner with a specific case. Postoperatively, the conversation between the faculty and learner is a *discussion* (D) to debrief on positive aspects of skill performance, as well as needed improvements in knowledge or skills as part of planning for future skill development. This framework encourages self-directed learning on the part of the resident, feedback on specific skills to the resident, and deliberate practice and feedback during the surgical experience.

Preoperative Briefing (B)

One simple way to maximize teaching for each surgical case is to use the BID model. The resident learns while planning the case, while doing the case, and by reviewing the case. By using this three-pronged approach to learning, maximum benefit from each case can be achieved, which improves educational efficiency, and helps address some of the problems outlined in the introduction to this chapter. Table 5.1 demonstrates an example of treating a patient with an intertrochanteric hip fracture with a cephalomedullary nail using the BID model. This is a fairly common fracture diagnosis and procedure in the United States, as well as a procedure that residents should be competent in performing under

TABLE 5.1 Operative teaching table

	Beginning resident (maximum assistance and supervision)	Mid-residency (moderate assistance and supervision)	Senior resident (minimal assistance and supervision)
Preoperative (preop plan as guide)	Resident to read about procedure preoperatively. Preoperative discussion of 1–2 surgical goals for resident. With X-rays, discussion of indications for surgery, including various options. Discussion of comorbidity. Classification of fracture. Discussion of consent and potential complications	With X-rays, discussion of indications for surgery, including comorbid factors. Include discussion of reduction techniques. Discussion of resident operative goals	Confirm indications for surgery, including comorbidities. Resident to explain reduction technique, implant, and potential difficulties foreseen preoperatively

TABLE 5.1 (continued)

	Beginning resident (maximum assistance and supervision)	Mid-residency (moderate assistance and supervision)	Senior resident (minimal assistance and supervision)
Operative	Attending present and scrubbed for most of the case. Conversation about optimal guide wire placement, basic reduction techniques. Demonstration of basic surgical principals	Attending present and scrubbed for all critical parts. Conversation and participation for critical parts of the case. Resident to perform parts of the case, with intervention by faculty when having difficulty. A smooth flow of differing parts of the case between faculty and resident should be the goal of allowing maximum resident participation but maintaining quality of care	Attending to be present for all critical portions of the case. For uncomplicated to moderately complicated fractures, the faculty member should not need to scrub in. Towards the end of training, the resident is expected to confirm their ability to perform this case

(continued)

TABLE 5.1 (continued)

	Beginning resident (maximum assistance and supervision)	Mid-residency (moderate assistance and supervision)	Senior resident (minimal assistance and supervision)
Postoperative	Attending to review with the resident the procedure, with discussion of what went well and what could be improved. Important to set goals for the next procedure of this type	Review with resident of case and the performance by the resident. Include goals for improvement. Discussion of postoperative plan, to include weight-bearing status, DVT prophylaxis, and antibiotics	Confirmation by resident of the postoperative plan to include the use of antibiotics, DVT prophylaxis, and weight-bearing status

the Accreditation Council of Graduate Medical Education (ACGME) Milestones (hip fracture).

For a preoperative discussion, a patient's history and physical are reviewed, diagnosis discussed, and an operative plan made. A preoperative plan, written by the resident and turned in to the attending prior to the surgery for review, is an excellent learning tool. A formal preoperative plan written out by the resident allows the resident to independently analyze the case, and allows the faculty to assess the resident's level of understanding prior to starting the case. This communication between faculty and resident is essential to maximizing the learning experience for each surgical case. This is particularly true of junior residents who may not have had exposure to this procedure. Reading about a procedure, followed by formulating a preoperative plan, which includes writing out the sequential steps, is a useful exercise for imprinting a procedure.

The preoperative plan is an educational tool that serves a number of important educational purposes including integrating anatomical knowledge, critical thinking, and importance of presurgical planning. While there are a number of ways to do this, the best way is one which allows robust discussion of the written preoperative plan that occurs between the faculty and resident. For fracture cases, it is best to draw out the anatomy, draw out the implant used, and then write the sequential steps in order of performance. Simple, low-tech drawings are the easiest to do as a learning exercise. This type of exercise can be done anywhere in the world, even under austere circumstances. Prior to the use of computers and preoperative templating of electronic X-rays, the simple drawings were often used. As a faculty member today, I am often presented with electronic X-rays which have an implant superimposed from a templating program. While this is a much easier exercise for resident to perform, there is often little critical thinking involved in formulating such a plan. Encouraging the residents to keep an electronic file of surgical plans is appealing to residents as these written surgical plans are useful for reference in later cases, and for when they embark in independent practice.

Depending on the level of the resident, the preoperative discussion should be done to ensure that the proper procedure is being planned, and a check of the equipment is needed, and the status of the patient with regard to preoperative clearance, consent, and need for blood. A junior resident will require more discussion to ensure that the patient has been properly cleared, the equipment is ready, and the procedure itself has been properly planned. Less double checking needs to be done by faculty once the resident is familiar with the routine for a given case. Preoperative clearance will become more automatic and expected of a resident as they advance through training. Educational goals should be set in the preoperative discussion. These educational goals should be used as guidance for the procedure. By verbal agreement, no more than 2–3 main goals for improvement should be sought for a particular case. Less experienced residents will perform less of the procedure when compared to a senior resident who is near graduation. When utilizing the operating room for teaching, performing simpler tasks of the procedure, followed by observation and seeing firsthand the more complex aspects of the case, is an important aspect of learning how to do a procedure. Building on the simpler experience to become more competent and have more autonomy during the case is the goal of teaching in the operating room. A mid-level resident who has participated in this procedure before will have more advanced goals for the procedure. Finally, the goal for a senior resident is to perform the procedure with minimal or no assistance from faculty.

Intraoperative Teaching (I)

Intraoperatively, the educational goals should follow what was discussed preoperatively. Outlining 1–3 goals prior to the onset of the procedure is a reasonable way to approach teaching in the operating room. Moulton et al. [2, 3] described surgical thought and behaviors as a transition back and forth between "automatic" and "effortful" [1, 2]. The automatic behavior is the accomplishment of the procedure or steps in the procedure in a routine manner. Most elective procedures in orthopaedic surgery are accomplished in this manner. More "effortful" behaviors are characterized by slowing down and concentrating on the unanticipated or more complex tasks. "Slowing down" to focus on the more critical teaching points of the case is extremely important for guidance and teaching. "Slowing down" will occur in areas where more time should be spent either with agreed-upon learning objectives for improvement during the case or in cases when unexpected events occur. Mastery of a surgical procedure will mean that the surgeon will accomplish the procedure automatically without giving the conscious thought to sequential steps. While some aspects of the case should be automatic, depending on the level of the resident, the areas which faculty and learner agree need work will be an effort of extra concentration allowing for possibly extra time to concentrate, receive feedback, and master the skill.

Debriefing (D)

Postoperatively, faculty and the resident should have a short discussion to debrief on what went well and what areas need additional training. Ideally, faculty should inquire as to what the resident felt went well and what areas for improvement still exist. Based on the resident's response, and faculty input, a future educational plan can be made for improving the resident's surgical skills. The postoperative discussion, therefore, becomes a mechanism where residents learn to identify gaps, elicit feedback, and develop an educational plan for future learning. Furthermore, the resident learns the case three times: before the case, doing the case, and debriefing the case. This maximizes educational efficiency.

In teaching, an important tenet is that the faculty member meet the resident where they are at and teach to their level. By identifying each resident's strengths and weaknesses, and skills can be built on throughout the rotation. This idea supports the resident working with a single faculty member for a rotation, allowing for the maximum amount of teaching to occur. With larger teams, and multiple faculty members, care must be taken to employ the BID technique each time, to know how to maximize the resident's experience and not just make the education too diffuse.

Operating Room Communication

Chen et al. [3–6] reported on interviews of nine attending surgeons and eight residents when observing operative interactions recorded by video between faculty and residents when performing one of eight common general surgery procedures [3, 5]. Both the attending surgeons and residents were then asked to review the videos and answer semistructured questionnaire. The authors found that there were three guiding behaviors demonstrated by faculty in the operating room which they characterized as teaching, directing, and assisting. *Teaching* was when the faculty demonstrated or described something new for the resident of the procedure. *Directing* behavior was when the resident was being guided verbally for an operative task. *Assisting* was when the faculty acts to facilitate the case, without prompting directions from the resident. An example of the latter would be to adjust a retractor as the resident is dissecting.

Roberts et al. attempted to identify verbal interactions that occurred in the operating room and categorize them as to the type of interaction being performed [1]. Four main types of interactions were described in this study. *Instrumental interactions* were used to move the procedure forward. In other words, this type of interaction was specific direction given by faculty member to move the case along in a timely manner. *Pure teaching interactions* were identified as those interactions in which the faculty provided enough context to improve the resident's understanding of the case. This type of interaction added to the resident's knowledge or was considered to help shape the resident's judgment.

A mixture of the previous two interactions was also noted. The use of *instrumental plus teaching interactions* provided guidance and provided a foundation for what was being accomplished at that point in the procedure. The last type of interaction that was noted was described as being "banter." This was considered by the authors to be conversation that was unrelated to the procedure. The authors went further to described "teachable moments" in which a faculty member noted an area of improvement, and described in real time a means to improve resident performance. On-the-spot, real-time, correction and improvement in resident performance is one of the most important facets of teaching in the operating room. In this study, the authors found that nearly half the interactions were "teaching" or "instrumental plus teaching."

In moving a case along, and facilitating progress, faculty need to assert themselves during the case to ensure that the procedure goes as is expected and that the teaching/learning experience is maximized.

Moulton et al. evaluated interactions between faculty and residents and how a faculty member controls the case to ensure that an appropriate balance between safety and education was maintained [2]. The authors interviewed 28 surgeons at 4 academic teaching hospitals, with 5 general surgeons being observed in the operating room. The authors were interested in evaluating how dynamics of the case proceeded when more difficult sections of the case were encountered which they referred to as "slowing down." They described how surgeons take direct control of the case when they perceive that the resident needs help or there is a more difficult section of the case. For more routine steps, they will often guide a resident through parts of the case, allowing for increasing autonomy as the resident gains the faculty confidence. Difficulties arise when the faculty and resident are "out of sync" with each other and do not see eye to eye on how the case should proceed. Additionally, the authors describe how faculty takes direct control of the procedure too late which results in either a less-than-optimal performance or a complication. The authors describe this as "skidding." Not trusting or having confidence in the residents' abilities does lead to too much control in which the resident is doing less than they are capable. The authors noted that bargaining was often done between residents and faculty in which doing more of the case was a reward for doing a job well, and less of the case as a punitive measure if the resident was perceived as doing less than expected.

Case Minimums?

While quality of education can influence the acquisition of skills, a certain amount of experience is needed to obtain a minimal proficiency for certain procedures. While perhaps no two cases are exactly the same, certain procedures lend themselves to repetitive practice. An example would be a primary total knee replacement or total hip replacement. Both procedures are part of the ACGME Milestones and are within the scope of practice for a general orthopaedic surgeon.

A learning curve to acquire minimal surgical skills or surgical skills similar to a standard of a practicing orthopaedic surgeon has been identified for procedures such as hip hemiarthroplasty, total knee and hip replacements, hip arthroscopy, cephalomedullary nailing for hip fracture, anterior hip replacement [7], hip resurfacing, use of a volar locking plate for distal radius fractures, as well as other procedures [7–10]. The outcomes used for each of these examples vary from time to completion of the procedure when compared to a practicing orthopaedic surgeon, to X-ray review, or comparison of patient outcomes.

When defining a content of capabilities for orthopaedic surgeons, the ability to perform competently those basic procedures included in the content is important. Procedures that need to be learned to a level of independent practice and competence are true for core orthopaedic procedures. Procedures that residents need to have familiarity, but only participate at an assistant level, would be true for specialty cases that require fellowship training. Work on defining core orthopaedic procedures for the general orthopaedic surgeon versus specialty orthopaedic procedures for the fellowship-trained surgeon has recently been presented [8].

Is there a role for case minimums of suitable common cases, knowing that a modicum of experience is required to be competent? Or should we move towards improving education and assessment towards a competency-based model in which the resident is deemed competent based on accomplishment of the procedure?

Organization for Education

Some aspects to produce optimal orthopaedic education are not well understood. Residencies have grown in size and scope over the last 70 years, and it is unclear on the best learning model. Two questions, important for any residency program, are the length of rotations and how teaching should be organized.

There is not a study comparing lengths of rotations and educational outcomes for residents. The length of rotations tends to be established by how many residents are there in the program or, in the case of interns, because of the scope of the PGY 1 year rotations need to be 4 weeks or one calendar month. Larger residency programs often have shorter rotation lengths after the PGY 1 than smaller ones. For example, in programs with eight residents and no overlap (or larger teams), the rotations would be approximately of 6 weeks' duration. Concerns about this short duration of the rotation, not allowing the faculty to know the resident as well and thus "not allowing them to do as much," can potentially be problematic. Within larger programs, scheduling with rotations is important to ensure adequate length as well as continuity with faculty. Smaller residency programs, such as those with three per year group, will have longer rotation lengths (4 months).

Which is better? While evidence supporting one over another for orthopaedic surgery residency remains sparse, some comments can be made. Larger programs with shorter rotations tend to allow for less length of time with a faculty member.

With shorter rotations, faculty members may have insufficient time to get to know the resident, provide feedback, and observe progression and education. With more frequent changes of residents, there can be less quality in the assessments. Likewise, with larger programs there tends to be a team associated with a particular service. This may mean that residents are exposed to multiple faculty members, who may not be able to get to know the individual resident very well, as with a preceptorship or apprenticeship model. Is it better for an individual resident to work with one or a few faculty members? In this author's opinion, it depends. There are different learning styles. Some residents may learn better in a mentorship model, working one on one with an attending, while other residents may learn better in a team model, when near-peer learning between residents is more available. The apprenticeship model tends to be the model for most orthopaedic fellowships today. Allowing for a period of time for the faculty to get to know the resident, provide feedback, and make improvements over time is a good model for learning surgical skills. With multiple faculty members, seeing varying techniques for a particular orthopaedic problem is appealing for some residents in terms of exposure to differing techniques for the same procedure. However, the resident will need to master a single technique, and then compare the other techniques to this standard. For the resident at a higher skill level, exposure to the multiple techniques may allow the resident to be better prepared to practice. Following this idea, having multiple faculty members provide multiple assessments for the resident may be stronger in terms of resident assessment from a statistical standpoint, but the assessments may not have enough quality to provide good feedback for the residents. Part of the match process in residents choosing a residency program is to assess the various models of surgical teaching, and choose a model that works best for them.

Surgical Simulation

The use of surgical simulation for teaching orthopaedic surgery is increasing. Changes which have occurred over the last two decades (resident duty hours, patient safety initiatives, and increased supervision requirements) have necessitated the ability to teach surgical skills outside of the operating room. Surgical simulation allows for practice and demonstration of surgical skills without compromising patient safety. Surgery is experiential, and allowing for multiple opportunities to practice in a safe environment allows a resident to gain experience without consideration of patient safety or operating room time.

As described above, procedures involve learning curves to become proficient, and surgical simulation allows for advancement of skills. Recent studies investigating the performance of knee and shoulder arthroscopy, cephalomedullary nail, pedicle screws, hip arthroplasty, and iliosacral screws all demonstrate improved proficiency with experience [7, 9–15].

Coughlin et al. developed a basic arthroscopic skill program based on low-fidelity models for triangulation and probing, grasping and transferring objects, tissue resection, as well as tissue suturing and arthroscopic knot tying [16]. The authors found that using these simple models could differentiate between the skills of medical students, interns, residents, and faculty. Not all orthopaedic simulators can do this. For example, sawbones models of simple fractures have an initial learning curve, but have a relatively low ceiling to obtain proficiency. Therefore, initial gains by novice doctors might occur, but no additional skills are gained for senior residents and faculty.

The American Board of Orthopaedic Surgery (ABOS) has initiated an intern surgical skill curriculum consisting of 17 modules [17]. These modules consist of motor skill education at a basic novice level. Topics include internal and external fixation, compartment syndrome, arthroplasty, basic suturing and knot tying skills, as well as bone-handling techniques and osteotomy.

Since 2013, all orthopaedic surgery residency programs must have the intern surgical skill program based on the ABOS modules. While it is too early to determine the results for this program, it does allow for earlier exposure of residents to orthopaedic surgical skill acquisition outside the operating room. Additionally, other changes of the PGY 1 year include 6-month orthopedic surgery, instead of the previous "up to three months" of orthopaedic surgery or subspecialty requirement prior to 2013. The intern surgical skill program, however, does require time and effort on the part of faculty to ensure that there is adequate supervision, as well as additional resources of space and equipment.

Teaching skills in a simulation laboratory, using cadaver or other simulators, does appear to help with acquiring skills. Faculty commit time to teaching sessions in order to have residents that enter the PGY2 year with better skills in the operating room [9, 18, 19]. As a department, developing the expectations for faculty participation in simulation events should be a priority. The purely teaching mission of faculty is extremely important and should be differentiated from time for assessment of the residents' performance. Teaching in a simulator environment tends to be less stressful, and allows the resident to perform an entire case without concerns of patient safety.

At the present time, simulation offers the benefit of allowing a resident to practice surgical skills within a safe environment. Low-technology simulators offer the most cost-effective instruction in this area. The use of simulation appears to benefit entry-level novice residents the most. Because of this, a structured approach for an intern-level simulation program seems best. Once the junior resident has obtained a sufficient level of proficiency, they are allowed to engage with the same procedures in the operating room.

Faculty Characteristics or Traits

A number of factors influence the ability to teach surgical skills. It is hard not to think of our own experiences and of those who taught us in medical school, residency, and fellowship. When did you learn the most? Who inspired you? Who taught you the most? Who did you like working with the best? The answer to these questions may not involve the same person.

Despite its importance, relatively few articles exist to help decide what faculty traits might contribute best to effective surgical education. Scheepers et al. reported on the responses of 622 attending physicians and 549 residents of surgical and nonsurgical specialties from the Netherlands [20, 21]. The authors used five personality domains to categorize the teaching faculty (consciousness, emotional stability, extroversion, agreeableness, and openness). The authors reported a positive correlation with extroversion and effectiveness of teachers across all specialties. The same group, reporting on faculty engagement and teaching effectiveness, found that more engaged teachers were better supervisors, and conscientiousness had the strongest correlation to teaching and patient care. The authors recommended that faculty development be individualized to improve faculty engagement and improve overall teaching.

Conclusion

Teaching operative skills is part of the responsibility of all faculty engaged in orthopaedic surgery resident education. How orthopaedic surgeons provide that teaching is highly variable. Because of increasing constraints of resident duty hours, operative time, and patient safety, maximizing efficiency with each teachable event for the best possible education for residents should be the goal. The use of the BID structured format to provide preoperative, intraoperative, and postoperative learning is the best way to get the most out of every procedure. Likewise, the use of simulation to provide multiple, repetitive practice for certain tasks on low-technology trainers is beneficial, particularly for those in the entry levels of residency, to allow for skill levels to develop at a minimal level before entering the operating room. Future educators will benefit from faculty development sessions oriented towards improving teaching skills.

References

1. Roberts NK, Williams RG, Kim MJ, Dunnington GL. The briefing, intraoperative teaching, debriefing model for teaching in the operating room. J Am Coll Surg. 2009;208(2):299–303.

2. Moulton CA, Regehr G, Lingard L, Merritt C, Macrae H. Operating from the other side of the table: control dynamics and the surgeon educator. J Am Coll Surg. 2010;210(1):79–86.
3. Moulton CA, Regehr G, Lingard L, Merritt C, Macrae H. 'Slowing down when you should': initiators and influences of the transition from the routine to the effortful. J Gastrointest Surg. 2010;14(6):1019–26.
4. Camp CL, Krych AJ, Stuart MJ, Regnier TD, Mills KM, Turner NS. Improving resident performance in knee arthroscopy: a prospective value assessment of simulators and cadaveric skills laboratories. J Bone Joint Surg Am. 2016;98(3):220–5.
5. Chen XP, Williams RG, Sanfey HA, Smink DS. A taxonomy of surgeons' guiding behaviors in the operating room. Am J Surg. 209(1):15–20.
6. Chen XP, Williams RG, Smink DS. Do residents receive the same OR guidance as surgeons report? Difference between residents' and surgeons' perceptions of OR guidance. J Surg Educ.71(6):e79–82.
7. de Steiger RN, Lorimer M, Solomon M. What is the learning curve for the anterior approach for total hip arthroplasty? Clin Orthop Relat Res. 2015;473(12):3860–6.
8. Kellam JF, Archibald D, Barber JW, Christian EP, D'Ascoli RJ, Haynes RJ, et al. The Core competencies for general orthopaedic surgeons. J Bone Joint Surg Am. 2017;99(2):175–81.
9. Bond W, Kuhn G, Binstadt E, Quirk M, Wu T, Tews M, et al. The use of simulation in the development of individual cognitive expertise in emergency medicine. Acad Emerg Med. 2008;15(11):1037–45.
10. Hoppe DJ, de Sa D, Simunovic N, Bhandari M, Safran MR, Larson CM, et al. The learning curve for hip arthroscopy: a systematic review. Arthroscopy. 2014;30(3):389–97.
11. Lonner BS, Auerbach JD, Estreicher MB, Kean KE. Thoracic pedicle screw instrumentation: the learning curve and evolution in technique in the treatment of adolescent idiopathic scoliosis. Spine (Phila Pa 1976). 2009;34(20):2158–64.
12. Magill P, Blaney J, Hill JC, Bonnin MP, Beverland DE. Impact of a learning curve on the survivorship of 4802 cementless total hip arthroplasties. Bone Joint J. 2016;98-B(12):1589–96.
13. Mayo BC, Massel DH, Bohl DD, Long WW, Modi KD, Singh K. Anterior Cervical Discectomy and Fusion: The Surgical Learning Curve. Spine (Phila Pa 1976).41(20):1580–5.

14. Nunley RM, Zhu J, Brooks PJ, Engh CA Jr, Raterman SJ, Rogerson JS, et al. The learning curve for adopting hip resurfacing among hip specialists. Clin Orthop Relat Res. 2010;468(2):382–91.
15. Nzeako O, Back D. Learning curves in arthroplasty in Orthopedic trainees. J Surg Educ. 2016;73(4):689–93.
16. Coughlin RP, Pauyo T, Sutton JC 3rd, Coughlin LP, Bergeron SG. A validated orthopaedic surgical simulation model for training and evaluation of basic arthroscopic skills. J Bone Joint Surg Am. 2015;97(17):1465–71.
17. ABOS Intern Surgical Skills Modules. ABOS.org/abos-surgical-skills-modules-for-pgy-1-residents.aspx.
18. Acton RD, Chipman JG, Lunden M, Schmitz CC. Unanticipated teaching demands rise with simulation training: strategies for managing faculty workload. J Surg Educ. 2015;72(3):522–9.
19. Kurahashi AM, Harvey A, MacRae H, Moulton CA, Dubrowski A. Technical skill training improves the ability to learn. Surgery. 2011;149(1):1–6.
20. Scheepers RA, Arah OA, Heineman MJ, Lombarts KM. How personality traits affect clinician-supervisors' work engagement and subsequently their teaching performance in residency training. Med Teach. 2016;38(11):1105–11.
21. Scheepers RA, Lombarts KM, van Aken MA, Heineman MJ, Arah OA. Personality traits affect teaching performance of attending physicians: results of a multi-center observational study. PLoS One. 2014;9(5):e98107.

Chapter 6
A Musculoskeletal Medicine Clerkship for Medical Students

Joseph Bernstein and Jaimo Ahn

Introduction

Musculoskeletal complaints represent one of the most common reasons people seek medical care—perhaps more than any other—yet the amount of time devoted to musculoskeletal topics in medical school is not commensurate to the burden of disease. Roughly 20% or more of primary care medicine visits are for problems related to the bones and joints, yet roughly only 2% of all curricular hours are devoted to this topic. In turn, surveys of young physicians indicate a lack of clinical confidence, and assessments of basic knowledge mastery have identified deficits [5, 6].

In response, the United States Bone and Joint Initiative (then known as the United States Bone and Joint Decade) started Project-100. This effort brought together various national stakeholder organizations, including the American Association of Orthopedic Surgeons, the National Board of Medical Examiners, and the Association of American Medical

J. Bernstein, MD (✉) • J. Ahn, MD, PhD
The Corporal Michael J. Crescenz VA Medical Center and
The University of Pennsylvania Perelman School of Medicine,
Philadelphia, PA 19104, USA
e-mail: joseph.bernstein@uphs.upenn.edu;
jaimo.ahn@uphs.upenn.edu

© Springer International Publishing AG 2018

P.J. Dougherty, B.L. Joyce (eds.), *The Orthopedic Educator*,
DOI 10.1007/978-3-319-62944-5_6

Colleges, among others, and through it has attempted to help and encourage medical schools to increase the emphasis schools place on this topic [2].

At the start of the USBJI's work, a survey of American medical schools showed that only about half of the schools had required instruction in musculoskeletal medicine [4]. Project-100 was so named because of its explicit goal of having 100% of American medical schools adopt a requirement for musculoskeletal instruction. A follow-up review 5 years later indicated that many more schools did indeed have required instruction, though for many, this instruction was placed in the preclinical years [1] (Table 6.1). As shown, the required clinical rotation was still a rarity.

In an ideal world, musculoskeletal medicine would have a prominent place in the preclinical and clinical curricula of all schools. Further, in this ideal world, instruction in musculo-skeletal medicine would transcend departmental lines: a community of musculoskeletal educators compromising not only orthopaedic surgeons, but also rheumatologists and physiatrists, anatomists, emergency physicians, general surgeons, internists, pediatricians, and many others, would come together to develop coherent curricula ideally adapted to the individual school's unique circumstances.

TABLE 6.1 Improvements in the rate of required musculoskeletal instruction in the USA, 2003–2011

Medical school curriculum requirements	2003	2011
Schools with a required preclinical course	42% (51/122)	79% (100/127)
Schools with a required clerkship	20% (25/122)	24% (31/127)
Any required instruction	53% (65/122)	83% (106/127)

Modified from Bernstein J, Garcia GH, Guevara JL, Mitchell GW: Progress Report: The Prevalence of Required Medical School Instruction in Musculoskeletal Medicine at Decade's End. Clinical Orthopaedics and Related Research 469(3), March 2011

In the meantime, it is not unreasonable for departments of orthopaedic surgery to take their own initiative and create course offerings that will fill the gap. After all, departments of orthopaedic surgery have the greatest concentration of musculoskeletal expertise (though certainly not a monopoly on it).

There are a few options for new courses in musculoskeletal medicine/orthopaedic surgery: a traditional fourth-year elective is orthopaedic surgery; a selective option as part of the surgery clerkship; and a free-standing required clerkship in musculoskeletal medicine/orthopaedic surgery.

The first option, the traditional fourth-year elective in orthopaedic surgery, is one in which a student spends about a month on the service, working alongside the resident teams. This is probably the easiest course to offer, though it is also likely the least helpful with regard to the greater aim of improving musculoskeletal education for all students. For one thing, an elective course by its nature will not be assuredly taken by all students. Also, by the time the fourth year has arrived, many students have committed to their chosen field, and thus a course then is likely to only "preach to the converted." Last, because many orthopaedic surgery electives serve the dual role of education-endeavor and audition-experience, they are likely to be particularly unrewarding for students not planning a career in orthopaedics. (In this auditioning environment, there is little pressure on faculty members to exert themselves in teaching, and the eager auditioning students, sharing the space with those participating just to learn, may be bit insufferable in the eyes of the latter.)

The selective option is typical in many schools. Traditionally, surgery was one of the major rotations of the clinical year, with students spending 3 months or so on the general surgery service. Over time, owing to increased specialization as well as decreased lengths of stay for hospital patients, these rotations have now devoted less time to inpatient general surgery, with greater opportunities for specialty rotations. Of the standard 12-week block, at least a few weeks are usually available for students to rotate on a specialty service—including not only orthopaedic surgery but also urology, neurosurgery, and plastic surgery, among others.

The selective experience is a little less intense that the fourth-year elective—not all students are auditioning—though it too is imperfect. For one thing, only a fraction of the class can take the selective. Also, because the selective is usually running within the surgery clerkship, the students' primary allegiance is to that course (and the final exam that might be waiting at the end of the 12-week block). It is also the case that this selective probably cannot cover the full gamut of musculoskeletal medicine, but rather emphasize those topics overlapping with surgery experience.

The other option is a required clerkship in orthopaedics. This option is not employed at many schools (for a variety of reasons), though it is one we have at our institution, the University of Pennsylvania. We currently offer a 1-week required clerkship for all students. We hope to share below a description of our course, not as much as an example for emulation—though that would be nice!—but to present some of the issues we've faced and why we have included certain things and omitted others. By so doing, we hope to identify some general principles and helpful suggestions that will allow a school to build its own coherent self-contained course.

Two Caveats

It is important to note two important caveats at the outset. The first is that a coherent clerkship experience cannot be "business as usual," if the baseline is simply to offer a tourist experience for the student. To be sure, a student interested in orthopaedic surgery as a career (the typical participant in an orthopaedic surgery course) will be highly motivated to please, and unduly acquiescent; these students traditionally have placed few demands on the residents and faculty. By contrast, students with other career plans will demand more attention. A new course, therefore, must be built with the understanding that more effort may be needed from the faculty. The second caveat is that a new course should not be undertaken on the assumption that it will necessarily improve recruitment to orthopaedic residency programs. It might [3], but that is gravy: in general, by the time a clerkship rolls around, students have already begun to shape their career plans. (Many students still have an open mind in the first year of school—and that's a strong argument for having orthopaedic surgeons participate in anatomy and other first-year courses.) These caveats sum to a simple recognition that offering any new or improved course will require orthopaedic surgery departments to do more, with few immediate rewards. Only with the larger perspective (of improving patient care and musculoskeletal outcomes) in mind does making this effort this make any sense.

The University of Pennsylvania Clerkship

Instruction at the University of Pennsylvania is divided among modules, but the general form of the four curriculum is 18 months of preclinical instruction; 12 weeks of clinical clerkships; and 18 months or more of additional study, covering a few additional requirements, electives, sub-internships, research opportunities, and others (about half of the students in any one entering class graduate more than 4 years after the start, many of whom earn a second degree).

Within the 18 months of preclinical instruction, there is no formal course in musculoskeletal medicine at the University of Pennsylvania, but, of course, musculoskeletal topics are covered in anatomy, pathophysiology, and other blocks.

The clinical year, which begins in January of the student's second year at the University of Pennsylvania, is devoted to ten required clerkships (Table 6.2). Orthopaedics 200, a required clinical rotation in orthopaedic surgery, is offered within the 3-month-long surgery block, but educationally independent of it. In addition to orthopaedics, students are required to spend 1 week in otorhinolaryngology and ophthalmology—together these are known as "the three Os"— and 1 week in anesthesia.

TABLE 6.2 Required clinical clerkships at the University of Pennsylvania

Clerkship	Duration (weeks)	Setting
Internal medicine	8	Inpatient
Family medicine	4	Outpatient
Obstetrics/gynecology	6	Combined in- and outpatient
Pediatrics	6	Combined in- and outpatient
Surgery	8	Combined in- and outpatient
Anesthesia	1	Inpatient
Ophthalmology	1	Combined in- and outpatient
Otorhinolaryngology	1	Combined in- and outpatient
Orthopaedic surgery	1	Combined in- and outpatient
Psychiatry	4	Combined in- and outpatient
Neurology	4	Inpatient
Emergency medicine	4	Emergency department

University of Pennsylvania has approximately 160 students, such that in each quarter 40 students are in the surgery block. Thirteen students then perform their specialty rotations in any given month. Orthopaedics 200 is then offered 1 week every month (12 times a year), carrying approximately 13 or 14 students in each iteration.

Although Orthopaedics 200 is technically a week-long course, the surgery didactics curriculum runs throughout the entire 12-week block—the students take a high-stakes shelf examination at the end of the 3 months—and half of every Friday is reserved for a general surgery education program that all 40 students participate in. Thus, there are 4 days available for clinical instruction (Table 6.3).

The basic organization of each of the 4 days controlled by orthopaedics is an educational conference in the morning, followed by clinical assignment from approximately 8 in the morning to 2 in the afternoon. At 3:00 p.m. the students

TABLE 6.3 Sample schedule of orthopaedics 200 at the University of Pennsylvania

	Monday	Tuesday	Wednesday	Thursday	Friday
6:15 AM	Orientation				Exam followed by exam review
6:30 AM conference	Orthopaedic surgery treatments	Orthopaedic surgery for the surgery shelf exam	Surface anatomy and physical exam of the hand	Grand rounds and education sessions	
730 am–2:30 pm	Clinical assignments	Clinical assignments	Clinical assignments	Clinical assignments	
3 pm Didactic seminar	Physical medicine	Fracture	Back pain	Arthritis	
6 pm–10 pm	Night call (optional)	Night call (optional)	Night call (optional)	Night call (optional)	

gather again for another educational conference just for them. Night call is optional. The morning educational conference on Monday, Tuesday, and Wednesday is specific for the students alone (that is, not for the residents as well), whereas on Thursday morning, our departmental educational day, the students join the residents for conference.

Because the students have such a short rotation, a choice must be made between depth and breadth: That is, do the students see different services each day, or stay with one for the entire week? We've tried both, and currently try to have most students maintain a relationship with the residents and faculty on a particular service for the week. Clearly there is a vast difference between, say, elective sports medicine arthroscopy and high-energy trauma fracture repair, or between adult and pediatric orthopaedics, and it would be nice for students to experience the vastness of orthopaedic surgery by sampling all of it. Nonetheless, sending students to four or more different services in a 4-day period invites scheduling difficulties and pedagogic incoherence.

The student-specific morning conferences are conducted by the chief resident, held apart from the morning conferences that the residents attend. The "slide deck" for these talks is kept on the department's server, and the responsibility for any one of these lectures is shared by any one of the eight chief residents, depending upon availability and interest.

The first lecture is called "Introduction to Orthopaedic Treatments." In this talk a review of what it is orthopaedic surgeons can do, and why they do it, is presented. There is a second talk entitled "Orthopaedic Surgery for the General Surgery Shelf Exam," covering those topics that are likely to be found on that high-stakes examination the students will be taking at the end of the block. There is a third talk on surface anatomy and physical examination of the hand. This was chosen primarily because the hand is easily exposed, and there are many nice anatomy correlations that can be presented. On Thursdays the students join the residents' education program. This is usually a basic conference for the residents, followed by a grand rounds lecture. The next 2 h is usually in the anatomy lab.

The afternoon didactic sessions include one on rehabilitation, led by a member of the Department of Physiatry. A second session is on fracture, including diagnosis, treatment, and basic biology. The Wednesday session is devoted to back pain and related physical examination topics and Thursday is dedicated to arthritis.

On Fridays students do not attend clinics. Half the day, as noted, is ceded to general surgery for its didactic program. In the afternoon students take an examination in orthopaedics, followed by a session in which the examination is reviewed. This examination is based on a self-learning module shared with the students at the beginning of the rotation, compromising approximately 50 questions in basic topics in musculoskeletal medicine. A sample of 5 of these 50 questions is selected verbatim for this exam. The booklet includes both the questions and the answers. The purpose of this examination is to motivate the student to read the booklet, and to make sure that at least this basic information is mastered. This examination is graded pass/fail.

The session on Friday is approximately 2 h in length. The students take the examination for the first 30 min—it usually doesn't take long, given that they have seen the questions in advance!—and the next hour-and-a-half is devoted to reviewing the questions, to make sure that the information was mastered. In addition, five related questions are presented to the students, in hopes of having a stimulating albeit brief discussion. A sample of a given test is shown in Table 6.4. The five questions are chosen arbitrarily, with the goal of rotating through most of the questions during the year.

Students are allowed (but not required) to take call, and are allowed (but not required) to submit a patient write-up and answer a few questions about that patient for consideration of the grade of Honors. Typically, about a third of the students elect to try for Honors, and approximately two-thirds of those attempting Honors earn it. (For students who elect to not take call, the course is pass/fail.)

TABLE 6.4 Sample Orthopaedics 200 examination at the University of Pennsylvania

Answer in writing	**To think about—no need to write; to be**
These will be graded	**Discussed when we review the test**
1. Tibia fractures might be complicated by a so-called compartment syndrome. What is a compartment syndrome and how is it prevented, diagnosed, and treated?	*What are some of the particular risks or dangers for patients with a tibia fracture complicated by compartment syndrome <u>in the setting of poly-trauma</u> (there are at least three and probably more)*
2. What are the four cardinal signs of osteoarthritis of the knee on plain radiographs?	*For each of the four cardinal signs of osteoarthritis, suggest how it may contribute to symptoms (or not); suggest how your hypothesis might be tested (or not)*
3. Provide a brief description of carpal tunnel syndrome: The chief complaints, examination findings, and treatment options	*At least to casual observation, carpal tunnel syndrome from overuse is considered a potentially work-related condition in BLUE (liberal) states but not in RED (conservative) ones. Provide an argument for and against the consideration of carpal tunnel syndrome as work related*
4. What is the function of the anterior cruciate ligament (ACL) in the knee? How is the ACL torn? Along those lines, why might it be the case that skiing-related ACL tears occur disproportionately after 2 pm?	*What else besides rank hypocrisy may prompt an attending surgeon who ordinarily berates you to "stop ordering tests and just examine the patient!" to order an MRI of a suspected ACL tear?*

TABLE 6.4 (continued)

Answer in writing	To think about—no need to write; to be
These will be graded	**Discussed when we review the test**
5. Describe the relationship between menopause and hip fracture risk. Describe the relationship between body mass and hip fracture risk	*Donald Trump (Penn '68) told Dr. Oz (Penn Med '86) that he is 6'3" and weighs 236 lb.—a BMI of 29—a perhaps dubious assertion. What are the musculoskeletal consequences of having a BMI >35 (a better estimate of the President's true state)*

Required Personnel

A successful course requires complete buy-in from the department chair and residency program director. Beyond that, the needed boots on ground, so to speak, include the teaching residents, the didactic faculty, and the course director(s).

At the University of Pennsylvania, we have an educational chief resident, who makes the clinical assignments, and presents the three resident talks (or ensures that others do). The educational chief resident is also available to solve problems regarding the clinical assignments. The didactic sessions in the afternoon are led by a member of the Department of Physiatry (Monday, rehabilitation), loyal and local volunteer alumni of our residency program (Wednesday, back pain), and a member of the Emeritus faculty (Thursday, arthritis). The course directors—the two authors here—present one of the afternoon sessions each (Tuesday, fracture; Friday, exam and review). In addition, the directors coordinate the schedule, grade the optional honors assignment, and participate in the medical school's committees for clerkship directors and related activities.

Knowledge, Skills, and Attitudes

Adult educational principles indicate that expectations and accountability for those expectations (as well as successful delivery of information, of course) drive learning. The actual content of expectations regarding knowledge, skills, and attitudes will differ based on the learner's baseline knowledge and the agreed-upon specifics that need to be tailored to the specific institution and situation. Nonetheless, explicitly stating these expectations sets the foundation for a successful course. Once determined, a mechanism of delivering the content will need to be formulated as well as methods for assessment. From feedback received over many years, it is clear that learners appreciate transparency and fairness for these expectations, delivery, and assessment.

Knowledge

Expectations: As an example we have used: "a core cognitive competency regarding the more common conditions encountered in musculoskeletal practice: arthritis; back pain; carpal tunnel syndrome; osteoporosis; fracture; and soft tissue injury, among others."

Delivery: Utilizing adult learning principles, we provided the students with content regarding a limited list of common musculoskeletal conditions that we expected them to master mostly on their own at their own pace (self-learning module), thus dictating basic facts to be learned while allowing for individual learning styles, and further content exploration based on interest. This is supplemented by basic morning lectures by residents (e.g., orthopaedic emergencies, content for the shelf examination) and late afternoon sessions with attendings (e.g., fractures, arthritis, imaging, and back pain), some of which is interactive in nature. Students also participate in approximately eight clinical sessions during the week rotations with a mixture of office/clinic and operating room experience. While we have attempted to make that experience thematically cohesive (trauma clinic with trauma OR), this represents "a tour" rather than systematic learning (like the didactic content) and is aimed more towards developing needed attitudes.

Assessment: Besides receiving immediate formative feedback regarding their answers during their didactic sessions, students are told that a summative examination will be given on the final day with topics directly from the self-learning module content that they are provided.

Skills

Expectations: As an example we have used "the ability to construct an anatomically directed hand examination (as a paradigm of all orthopedic examinations)."

Delivery: Although the teaching of examination of several extremity joints and the spine would be ideal as well as specific treatment skills (reduction, splinting, casting), we decided to use a specific joint as a paradigm so as to work within the framework of the course. (We also knew that shoulder and spine examinations were covered in the family medicine clerkship.) Teaching of this content is best executed in small groups with a dominant hands-on component, perhaps using each other models with immediate feedback. This is supplemented by observation/participation in the clinic and OR (as well as optional "call" with residents) although, again, these modes remain nonsystematic in a short time frame and emphasize attitudes instead. In addition, because "required" course time is scarce, faculty have worked in conjunction with student leader-teachers to organized near-peer skill sessions related to physical examination, casting, splinting, etc.

Assessment: Feedback is almost completely formative with real-time comments to guide improvement until competence is obtained. Summative evaluation such as the use of an OSCE or a specific skill test (instructor or mechanically/electronically administered) has not been feasible within a 1-week course; however, the development of efficient and effective methods for summative evaluation and feedback will enhance learning in the future.

Attitudes

Expectations: As an example we have used "an appreciation for the impact of musculoskeletal disease on the happiness, function and well being of patients; an appreciation of the role of pain as an impediment to happiness and function; an appreciation of what doctors of musculoskeletal medicine can (and cannot) offer their patients."

Delivery: This is the most difficult of the goals to teach (and assess). By educating and discussing our goals as teachers with residents and attending staff, our goal has been to convey this content through the use of all of our delivery mechanisms including knowledge through the self-learning module, didactic teaching (faculty instructors and near-peer leaders), clinic/OR sessions, call, and further self-directed learning. It is perhaps by improving in this domain that we can attract further diversity and increasingly engender affective excellence within orthopaedics.

Assessment: We do not know of a valid method of assessment for this goal. As a proxy, however, we do offer an "Honors" grade for those inclined to delve into the "appreciation" that we conjure. Interested students are incentivized to take call, and provide a thoughtful write-up based on evaluating a patient in order to receive the superlative grade resulting in a better appreciation for our field and what we offer our patients.

Implementing a New Course

Departments of orthopaedic surgery that are planning a new course—of any variety or duration—can likely count on the education office to articulate the school's requirements and to make sure that these are met. Beyond that, we suggest that some additional steps be taken. These, and their rationale, are shown in Table 6.5.

TABLE 6.5 Planning steps for a new course in orthopaedic surgery

Step	Rationale
1. Assess your resources and commitments: Ensure that you have the wherewithal to deliver	Resources and commitments are the rate-limiting step. As much as one may like the notion of having a new course, the opportunity costs may be prohibitive. Don't even think of proposing a course for which new resources must be created
2. Articulate a mission statement: Define what are you trying to achieve, given your resources.	Because there are typically so few courses, a course that does anything is likely to be (seen as) an advance; but a course that does "anything" might be incoherent and short-lived.
3. Create a plan for evaluation: Recognize when you have met your goals—or not	This is self-evident, but may be overlooked. Also, a system of evaluation distinct and apart from the school's system of evaluation may be helpful
4. Cultivate your replacement	"The cemeteries are full of indispensable men"—Clemenceau

Conclusion

Schools looking to add teaching experiences in musculoskeletal medicine and orthopaedic surgery can consider a traditional fourth-year elective, a selective within the surgery clerkship, or free-standing musculoskeletal medicine/orthopaedic surgery course. Yet while those may be the choices currently available in 2017 at most schools, it is highly likely that in the coming years there were will be a complete revamping of organization of medical school, including a reclamation of the fourth year (which is currently devoted to residency applications, and courses of insufficient rigor). When that happens, there will be opportunities for implementing not only new courses but also new types of courses.

And just as cities that had "shovel-ready" projects were more likely to receive federal grants of cash under the American Recovery and Reinvestment Act of 2009 (the so-called stimulus spending bill), departments that have educational plans ready for review are more likely to be blessed by curriculum committees with grants of time. It is with that thought in mind—that major reform may be coming, and musculoskeletal medicine should be part of it—that faculties should consider what they hope to achieve in musculoskeletal medicine education, and how to do it.

References

1. Bernstein J, Garcia GH, Guevara JL, Mitchell GW: Progress report: the prevalence of required medical school instruction in musculoskeletal medicine at decade's end. Clin Orthop Relat Res 469(3):895-897 2011
2. Bernstein J, Alonso DR, DiCaprio M, Friedlaender GE, Heckman JD, Ludmerer KM. Curricular reform in musculoskeletal medicine: needs, opportunities, and solutions. Clin Orthop Relat Res. 2003;415:302–8.
3. Bernstein J, DeCaprio MR, Mehta S. The relationship between required medical school instruction in musculoskeletal medicine and application rates to orthopaedic surgery residency programs. J Bone Joint Surg. 2004;86:2335–8.
4. DeCaprio MR, Covey A, Bernstein J. Curricular requirements for musculoskeletal medicine in American medical schools. J Bone Joint Surg. 2003;85:565–7.
5. Freedman KB, Bernstein J. The adequacy of medical school education in musculoskeletal medicine. J Bone Joint Surg. 1998;80A(10):1421–7.
6. Freedman KB, Bernstein J. Educational Deficiencies in Musculoskeletal Medicine. J Bone Joint Surg. 2002;84:604–8.

Chapter 7
Orthopaedic Resident Assessment: Measuring Skills in Both Knowledge and Technical Skills

S. Elizabeth Ames, Nathaniel Nelms, and Donna Phillips

S. Elizabeth Ames, MD (✉)
Associate Professor and Program Director Department of Orthopaedics and Rehabilitation, The Robert Larner, MD College of Medicine, University of Vermont, 95 Carrigan Drive, Robert T. Stafford Hall, 4th Floor, Burlington, VT 05405, USA

Assistant Professor Department of Orthopaedics and Rehabilitation, The Robert Larner MD College of Medicine University of Vermont, 95 Carrigan Drive, Burlington, VT 05405, USA
e-mail: elizabeth.ames@med.uvm.edu

N. Nelms, MD
Associate Professor and Program Director Department of Orthopaedics and Rehabilitation, The Robert Larner, MD College of Medicine, University of Vermont, 95 Carrigan Drive, Robert T. Stafford Hall, 4th Floor, Burlington, VT 05405, USA
e-mail: Nathaniel.Nelms@uvm.edu

D. Phillips, MD
Clinical Professor Orthopaedic Surgery and Pediatrics, Chief Pediatric Orthopedic Surgery Bellevue Hospital, Bellevue Hospital, 462 1st Avenue CD489, New York, NY 10016, USA
e-mail: Donna.Phillips@nyumc.org

© Springer International Publishing AG 2018
P.J. Dougherty, B.L. Joyce (eds.), *The Orthopedic Educator*,
DOI 10.1007/978-3-319-62944-5_7

Introduction

Graduate medical education has traditionally been steeped in experiential, workplace-based learning. Residents are taught and supervised by faculty with different levels of expertise, and frequently only work with senior residents for short periods of time. It has always been true that faculty must be able to model, teach, assess, and remediate orthopaedic residents and generally we have done this well. Chapter 3 outlines the shift to competency-based education; this is familiar ground as we have always been about creating and certifying competence in surgical trainees. In terms of assessment, though, this is a whole new world.

Most of us have been trained in an environment of summative assessment—pass/fail decisions to determine whether a minimum criterion has been achieved. Educational standards now require a transformational shift in curriculum and assessment measures. The evolution today is towards formative education as we transition to competency assessment. This evolution is associated with a need to respond to broad national educational goals and accreditation requirements, as well as continuing to meet evolving specialty content. Ultimately we need to develop a solid program of tools and educational structures designed to assess and inform the learner as their skills develop with the ultimate goal of both knowledge and technical improvement.

Our challenge is to adjust to all of these changes without having had exposure to them in our own education. Meaningful training in resident assessment must meet the new metrics. The goal is defined—measuring the educational level of the learner, providing actionable feedback, and ultimately ensuring the learner transitions from novice to "competent." The challenge to orthopaedic surgery programs is understanding which type of assessments are needed, establishing a real and measurable definition of what competence is for our specialty, and choosing the right tools to assess it. The purpose of this chapter is to consider the history of resident assessment, to present the state of the art of what is available currently, and create a resource that encourages faculty to look forward into how things can be done differently as orthopaedic training continues to evolve.

Resident Assessment Overview: Competency-Based Assessment

All assessment tools and systems represent some form of compromise. The choice (and use) of any system will vary depending on a program's needs and staff. Assessment systems can and should include multiple measures or tools that capture faculty opinions and provide feedback to the residents. The choice of type and number of tools within a resident assessment system are completely up to the individual program with two exceptions. The ACGME's Next Accreditation System mandates reporting milestone outcomes and individual case volumes through the case log system. A review of these two systems and suggestions for other assessments follows.

Milestones are an example of a reporting system that requires direct assessment of residents. Orthopaedics was one of the first specialties involved in the creation of milestones, and many educational leaders within the specialty contributed to the effort. Our milestones are known for being particularly numerous, but are well focused within each area of the specialty. The tools themselves are relevant and useful. The key for each subspecialty is developing a reliable, consistent, and useful process for implementing the milestones to track and report educational outcomes. One specific challenge is to maintain a consistent reporting system in a busy clinical world. The quality of the assessments will vary if the program, faculty, or residents find the reporting tool overly burdensome or not particularly useful [1]. Techniques to avoid needless burden while maintaining utility are being explored in the UK where a mandatory work-based assessment system exists [2]. The influence of the work environment also needs to be recognized with variation in social factors, competing tasks, and fatigue [3]. Variability is part of any clinical rating scheme, and significant faculty development should be implemented to reduce rater variability with the milestones.

Education of both faculty and residents is required to appropriately measure milestones. Faculty and resident perceptions significantly influence the utility of any assessment system; milestones provide an opportunity to give constructive feedback which may be best delivered during a face-to-face conversation. The goal of milestones is to provide actionable feedback to the resident; this is lost if milestones are assigned without direct discussion behind the assigned score. Comparative data for the first years of milestone implementation is now available from the ACGME (http://www.acgme.org/What-We-Do/Accreditation/Milestones/Overview) and specialty specific data will be available in 2017.

The other required ACGME report is the evaluation of the operative cases completed by each resident per year. The standards set by the orthopaedic RRC are considered case minimums that describe exposure, and do not necessarily document technical competence. This report can and should be considered a reflection of the educational design of a residency program and ultimately allows comparison with other programs. Attention to details of the educational process is important to have this data accurately reflect the learning model. Comparative data between programs is available as part of the annual residency review process.

Milestones and case logs demonstrate the benefits of adding formative assessment to the traditional summative model as they record a resident's progress towards competence. The milestones depend on direct faculty supervision and link technical skill development to episodes of learning. Hence faculty development plays an important role in both these assessments. It is important to note that evaluators are more likely to use the full range of available scores when the scale is referenced to a scale of competence rather than assigning a score [4] referenced only against instructor expectations. Competency-based assessment can be referenced to clear final educational goals. This will have improved validity, particularly when multiple observers use the same scale accompanied by a periodic monitoring, assessment, and committee review process [5]. This is the model behind the Clinical Competency Committee and other ACGME reporting structures.

Finally, residency programs need to honestly assess issues such as a reluctance to fail trainees. There are several strong factors that contribute to this [6]. These factors include lack of confidence among faculty in their ability to detect failure, lack of documentation to support failure, a lack of direct communication with the resident about the issues, and a real or perceived lack of ability to remediate a failure. These issues can be addressed by including more points of assessments during resident training and avoiding reliance on just a few high-stakes evaluations. Work-based assessment is best done on multiple occasions by multiple evaluators. Developing this sort of structure, with points of view from many angles, creates a robust view of trainee progress, and the opportunity to focus on achieving optimal competency in all residents.

Resident Assessment Overview: Testing and Metrics

There are two traditional testing methods within orthopaedic surgery—the Orthopaedic In-Training Examination (OITE) administered by the AAOS and the two-part written and case-based examination administered by the ABOS. The ABOS and ACGME/RRC for Orthopaedic Surgery also mandated the introduction of simulation training for the PGY-1 in 2013. Fully developed modules are available on the ABOS website and will not be reviewed here.

Objective assessment is a challenge. Standardized written examinations continue to have value for both individual resident assessment and programmatic design. The OITE is a multiple-choice examination of approximately 275 questions across multiple subject areas including orthopaedic basic science. It is now administered to over 4000 orthopaedic residents worldwide, and was the first in-training examination created by any specialty. It is not administered in a standardized way nor required of residencies and, therefore, is not directly related to subsequent certification testing. It is widely used, however, and as it has developed the reporting has become much more robust with stratification by program type (allopathic or osteopathic) and year in training. It does allow the individual resident to compare his or her progress relative to their peers in the same year of training, and a program to track overall performance by subject content. It also has some utility as an approximation for relative performance on future certification exams.

There is literature that explores both the correlation between the OITE and other exams and the methods that current orthopaedic residents use to prepare. In 2013 Evaniew et al. surveyed both program directors and residents in North America [7]. Focus on preparation, importance cited by the program, and reported hours spent preparing were predictive of higher OITE scores in comparison to others in the same year in training. References cited for test questions primarily come from journal articles (74%) or textbooks (26%) in recent studies [8, 9]. This may be shifting with the development of electronic resources [10]. Individual program standards and approaches to this test vary.

Studies have explored the relationship between OITE scores and ABOS Part 1 pass rates [11–13]. The exams are designed, administered, and scored differently and ABOS is a pass/fail exam but percentiles are reported to programs. Ponce et al. looked at subsection scores over 10 years at one program and found that the areas with greater content representation did correlate with ABOS performance most notably in PGY3 and PGY4 [14]. They and others have concluded that the OITE can be used to help identify residents at risk for failing ABOS Part 1.

The larger question is how a program should respond to a low OITE score. The authors' opinion is that every program should decide on an overall target metric relevant to historical performance data, and the standards should be clear to the residents. The one clear point is that poor performance often reflects a struggling resident and early, customized exploration and intervention are useful.

Nonoperative Skill Assessment:

Evaluation of resident skills in the clinic has traditionally consisted of an apprenticeship model; relationships in this model are deep with significant time spent together. Dedicated teaching rounds are not as common in orthopaedic programs today, which is one indication that times are changing. Historically verbal formative feedback was mostly used to correct deficiencies, and formal written evaluation was not very instructive. At best, some verbal formative feedback was provided to the learner and one or two written evaluations were given to the program director during the course of a rotation. Better optimization of the feedback piece is of great importance for implementation of competency-based education.

The current system of medical education can make it difficult to sustain face-to-face interaction. We still spend significant time face to face with a resident during an operative case, but the clinical environment has other challenges. An orthopaedic resident's ability to diagnose and manage patients in a nonoperative setting such as clinic or hospital rounds is as important as their operative skills but has become difficult to teach and assess. Residents have varying interactions with multiple faculty members often across different medical systems. Time spent being directly observed is limited by clinical demands on both parties. Tools to assess these skills are beginning to develop.

Clinical skills such as history taking, physical exam, and informed consent are best assessed through multiple types of evaluations. These can include oral and written examinations, case-based discussions, work-based assessments, and simulated patient encounters [15, 16]. The use of multiple types of evaluations is of particular value as no single task exists independently in the real world. It is important to avoid deconstructing tasks into a checklist of achievements—a checklist approach does not equate to true clinical competency [17]. These challenges are met by direct observation which is a comfortable assessment tool for surgeons. There are both specific tools and systematic approaches that apply to direct observation.

Several tools are available to structure the evaluation of clinical skills. The goal is to provide real-time feedback to the learner in a constructive way while simultaneously building the groundwork for a summative assessment. Several tools demonstrate validity and are applicable to the evaluation of orthopaedic residents including the Mini-Clinical Evaluation Exercise (Mini-CEX), Clinical Assessment and Management Examination Outpatient (CAMEO), and the Ottawa Clinic Assessment Tool (OCAT). They are also reasonably easy to incorporate into a faculty development program. Each is described and referenced below.

The Mini-CEX is validated and is the most widely used tool for assessment of focused clinical encounters. The evaluation includes four measures: history taking, physical examination, clinical judgment and synthesis, and humanism. Each is scored on a point scale from unsatisfactory to superior with an option for any category to score as "insufficient contact to judge." The original CEX evaluation was based on in-depth observation by faculty of a resident's comprehensive single-patient evaluation [18]. The Mini-CEX has been widely adopted by multiple specialties and has demonstrated validity [18–22].

The CAMEO is a modified version of the Mini-CEX designed to evaluate residents working specifically in a surgical clinic [23]. A 5-point scale is used to evaluate the following domains: test ordering and understanding, diagnostic acumen, history taking, physical examination, communication skills, and overall performance. Evaluators also note the chief complaint, presumptive diagnosis, and difficulty of the case for each assessment. The CAMEO is recognized as a valid form of resident assessment, and the American Board of Surgery (ABS) requires general surgery residents to have documented evaluations of observed patient encounters with either the Mini-CEX or the CAMEO. Both of these tools are available on the ABS website (http://www.absurgery.org/default.jsp?certgsqe_resassess).

The Ottawa Clinic Assessment Tool (OCAT) is similar in format to the CAMEO, but has a few important features that make it an attractive option for orthopaedics [4]. The OCAT is based on an entire day of clinic instead of a single observed encounter, and was specifically designed for a busy surgical clinic where a faculty member may observe a resident in several domains, without necessarily directly observing an entire patient encounter. There are nine areas of global assessment, a procedural skill question, a yes/no professionalism question, a yes/no for the ability to manage a clinic independently at a generalist level, and two open-ended questions regarding specific examples of something that went well and something that could use improvement. The areas of global assessment include history, physical exam, case presentation, differential diagnosis, management plan, communication skills, documentation, collaboration, and time management. Each of these areas is graded on a 1–5 scale relative to the goal of readiness for independent practice.

The basic premise behind most of these modern evaluation tools is the concept of Entrustable Professional Activities described by Ten Cate in 2005 and reviewed recently [24]. This idea allows competencies to be operationalized and measured in a work environment, and reflects the need to make a judgement about a resident's independence that is inherent in orthopaedic education. Assessment systems referenced to a level of competence that allows entrustable activities to occur have distinct relevance to orthopaedic education as long as reference points are relatively clear. On an entrustment scale like the OCAT, a resident can be assessed as able to make management decisions with some staff direction (3/5). A score of 5/5 represents that the supervision from the attending was not required. This offers advantages over the more traditional poor to excellent numerical scales which can be interpreted and used differently by different raters—for example, one rater might compare a resident to the "usual resident at that training level," another to current peers, and another to what is expected for graduation. The ultimate goal of a competency-based assessment system is to reflect progressive independence as defined by the vast majority of faculty.

Direct Observation

The ACGME requires that residency programs teach and assess trainees in six core competencies: medical knowledge, patient care, interpersonal and communication skills, professionalism, systems-based practice, and practice-based learning and improvement. It is challenging to provide specific feedback to trainees with respect to these, and the last four are difficult to assess without direct observation. It is also true that the nontechnical competencies are crucial to providing patient-centered care (PCC) which is dependent on excellent communications skills and professionalism [25, 26]. The American Academy of Orthopaedic Surgeons (AAOS) developed a communications skills workshop focused on orthopaedic-specific scenarios [27, 28]. Unfortunately, it cannot be assumed that teaching and modelling communication skills and professionalism in a classroom results in incorporation of those skills into actual practice. Implementation of a direct observation program has significant advantages in these areas.

Direct observation programs require tools. A systematic approach with a checklist individualized to a residency structure currently exists in orthopaedic and other training programs. A user-friendly broad electronic platform assists with reporting to both residents and administration. Programmatic structure and faculty skill development are required as with any assessment system. The scope of skills to be assessed is broad—options include elements of a clinical history, physical exam, and review of data such as radiographs. The scope can be tailored to the specific rotation or environment which improves efficiency and relevance. System-based tasks such as discussion of surgical risks, indications, and patient safety awareness such as handwashing before and after contact with the patient can be added. Overall impressions and real-time comments can both be incorporated. Trainee self-assessment prior to reviewing the faculty evaluation may also be included.

The challenge in this type of program is in creating it to match specific goals while providing complete assessment.

Once tailored to programmatic needs the implementation is efficient. The assessments are performed by trained observers in the clinic or on inpatient rounds and can be part of usual patient care or purely scored by a dedicated observer. The assessor accompanies the trainee into the exam room, and is introduced to the patient as an observer of the resident for educational purposes. The encounter proceeds as it normally would between resident and patient. The observation can be for all or some of the encounter. The observer reviews the encounter with the resident for about 5 min immediately following the patient visit to debrief. At this point the resident is provided specific, structured feedback using a checklist as a guide.

Observing each trainee at least four times a year is recommended for early detection of deficiencies and appropriate coaching and tracking. The summary of the data for the entire training group can be used as a needs assessment to monitor the residency curriculum. The Clinical Competency Committee (CCC) can use this data to support the assessment of milestones. Individual data can be reviewed with the trainee during biannual reviews. Residents who demonstrate deficiencies in one or more competency domains can be scheduled for more frequent observations.

One author's (DP) experience can be cited as an example. This program emphasizes the importance of nontechnical competencies as crucial for safe patient care and therefore meets many external quality goals. The resident is provided with immediate feedback regarding the tools they will need to develop a practice with high patient satisfaction. The ACGME core competencies are assessed in the outpatient setting. The ability to complete a history and physical examination is observed (patient care and medical knowledge). Communications skill assessment includes the skills taught in the AAOS communications skills workshop [28]. Professionalism concerns such as fatigue, professional appearance, and accountability are documented. Any discussion of cost containment (systems-based practice) is documented. If the entire encounter has been observed the medical record is reviewed (systems-based practice) for internal consistency, documentation of clinical reasoning, cut-and-paste errors, and completeness and accuracy. Practice-based learning is part of the assessment process. Trainees are asked to self-assess—to recognize skills that were effective, and identify challenges or portions of the encounter that could be improved. Faculty observers determine if the resident is conscious of skills they perform well, and skills that need to be further developed [29].

A shorter checklist is used for observing residents rounding on multiple inpatients, focusing on the expected communications skills, patient safety, privacy, and work in interprofessional teams. The resident describes the observer's role to the patient; their ability to clearly present this—even if it is the attending surgeon—is key. Fortunately, the use of scribes and other medical paraprofessionals has made this an easily acceptable part of patient life. At the end of rounds, the resident's handoff skills are observed and assessed for efficiency and accuracy which helps meet direct ACGME requirements.

Direct observation in a clinical or hospital setting is clearly not something most faculty educators were exposed to during their training. Programs of any size or complexity can develop a structured direct observation program as long as both faculty and trainees are made familiar with the purpose and clear, consistent faculty development is provided. A well-organized, 90-min workshop in small groups of up to eight faculty members has been sufficient to successfully launch a program in both orthopaedics and in other surgical specialties [30]. Early results from over 400 observations of 63 residents in outpatient clinics and hospital rounds have demonstrated that trainee skills cannot be predicated based on their reputation among attending surgeons, their observed skills in conferences, or the operating room. Trainees with strong leadership skills within the residency group or with strong technical skills may have limited skills in patient encounters, and vice versa. Consistent observations with many faculty participating and strong support from department leadership have resulted in a culture change whereby observations are an expected part of resident experience. Direct, structured feedback in the workplace has been valued by house staff.

Surgical Skill Assessment

The mastery of particular surgical skills requires ongoing formative assessment and feedback in near real time. Surgical skill evaluation is important for ongoing resident development, and ultimately forms the basis for documenting surgical competency. This is also a place where orthopaedic faculty tend to feel more comfortable, a form of "I know it when I see it." The challenge for orthopaedic attendings completing the assessment loop is to understand where the resident is in preparation for the case, to allow progressive responsibility, and to do all this efficiently in the setting of clinical stressors. This is the concept of actionable feedback—intervening as an instructor when the stakes are high and the path is clearly defined. The reward is that providing ongoing information to residents in near real time allows the learner to focus their efforts towards mastery of particular skills—and mastery in one small area is rewarded by improved ability to learn the next.

Assessment of resident surgical skills remains largely the purview of orthopaedic faculty. Residents should be given appropriate responsibilities in a gradual and progressive manner. Clear instructions and defined expectations help set goals for skill acquisition and this starts with procedure planning. Face-to-face discussion clarifies the goals of the procedure and helps focus later evaluation. It also allows faculty an assessment of where the resident is if a long-standing relationship is not available as is often the case in the current medical environment.

There are processes that can help balance some of the challenges in medical education today. Handoffs between faculty members can communicate general observations on the progress of a resident's operative skills and can maintain teaching flow as one rotation ends and another begins. It is also apparent that the skills needed during a resident's career may be very different than those needed today. This makes it all the more important to train surgical residents to be adaptive and willing to continue deliberate practice through self-awareness and engagement of communities of experts [31].

Traditionally evaluation systems have included informal day-to-day interactions and end-of-rotation written evaluations reviewed by the Program Director (PD). The summary of collective reports is used by the PD to certify the surgical competency of the individual. There are multiple broad reporting metrics for case numbers and these are useful and mandatory forms of assessment. There are also opportunities to incorporate a rubric or systematic rating scales to structure evaluations of technical skills, and some of those are readily available.

The Structured Technical Skills Assessment Form (STSAF) was an early effort created to assess general surgical skills [32]. This form rates resident abilities specific to the procedure such as proper patient positioning, equipment preparation, incision placement, and some technical aspects of the procedure. The STSAF also included a global rating for respect for tissues, the use of assistants, instrument names, following sterile technique, working well with others, and keeping the operation flowing. This tool provides inter-rater reliability and the ability to differentiate between residents by training level.

The Objective Structured Assessment of Technical Skills (OSATS) was developed at the University of Toronto in the late 1990s with the components of a task-specific checklist and a global rating scale [33]. It was initially developed for use as a bench simulation-type examination and has since been applied to the evaluation of intraoperative skills; as of now there is not strong evidence to support its use in that form for high-stakes exams [34, 35]. A secondary concern is that general tools do not assess the final result of quality of the surgical outcome as demonstrated in an intra-articular fracture reduction model in 2016 [36].

The OSATS global rating scale (GRS) was the next step towards intraoperative assessment. This tool contains a 5-point Likert scale assessing respect for tissue, time and motion efficiencies, instrument handling and knowledge, flow of the procedure, use of assistants, and general preparatory knowledge. The GRS has been compared to other validated procedure-specific evaluation tools such as Global Operative Assessment Of Laparoscopic Skills (GOALS) and found to have near-perfect correlation, which has led to investigations as to whether procedure-specific evaluation tools are needed [37, 38].

In 2007 Doyle described the Global Rating Index for Technical Skills (GRITS) which has a format and content like OSATS but adds specific skills like camera depth perception and endoscopic dexterity. The Basic Arthroscopic Knee Skill Scoring System and the Arthroscopic Surgical Skill Evaluation Tool (ASSET) are orthopaedic equivalents [39, 40]. The ASSET uses a Likert scale ranging from novice to expert in the categories of safety, field of view, camera dexterity, instrument dexterity, bimanual dexterity, flow of procedure, quality of procedure, and autonomy. It also includes a task-specific checklist for diagnostic arthroscopy and has demonstrated reliability and validity in expert review. Tools for other skills such as managing a fractured radius are also under development.

In 2012 the Ottawa Surgical Competency Operating Room Evaluation (O-SCORE) was developed by Gofton et al. [41] This tool assesses pre-procedure plan, case preparation, knowledge of procedural steps, technical performance, visual-spatial skills, post-procedure plan, case efficiency and flow, and communication and adds a single yes/no question as to whether the resident could perform the procedure independently. The O-SCORE assesses the learner relative to the final skill competency goal and not relative to resident peers or training level. The scoring scale for faculty is in a familiar voice ("I had to do most of the procedure" vs. "I did not need to be there".). One open-ended response is also required for a specific aspect that went well, and one suggestion for improvement. The O-SCORE has demonstrated validity for the first 4 years of residency; it loses discrimination ability between PGY4 and PGY5 levels [42]. A recent modification includes a 5-point summary scale which added additional value [43].

Technological advancements will help manage the time crunch of the operating environment. Tools like the four-item Zwisch scale can also be easily adapted to an electronic evaluation platform. The Zwisch scale is a behaviorally anchored scale that grades the degree of guidance the attending surgeon provides to the trainee during the most critical portion of the procedure [43]. Levels from "Show and Tell" to "Passive Help" to "Active Help" to "Supervision Only" describe the resident's involvement. This was validated like the O-SCORE to be strongly discriminative in PGY1–4 but less useful in the PGY4–5 transition. The electronic format was easy to use with a 92% response rate supporting the possibility of both improved and more longitudinal resident assessment data.

A very similar tool is under investigation by the ABOS for assessing technical skills in orthopaedic residency. Multiple programs are piloting a summative scale in 2017 that matches expected PGY skills at key points in the course of training. The goal is to expand this to a wide variety of residency training programs on an electronic platform, which has not yet been reported in any specialty. The three categories are novice (PGY1–2), low intermediate (PGY2–3), and high intermediate (PGY3–4) with five to seven descriptive skills in each category. The three overarching descriptions with respect to overall function are "attending surgeon provides maximum assistance," "attending surgeon provides significant assistance and direction," and "attending provides modest assistance and direction," each associated with specific technical skill-level demonstrations. Operative assessment can also be done with technical tools such as video review of procedures, tracking of hand motions, and instrument pressure monitors [44, 45, 46]. There may be a great future to these types of technologies at least in simulation laboratory learning, but currently these types of systems are not widely available and may not in their current version provide value given the cost.

Challenges

An effective system for the assessment of operative skills requires faculty education. This has been recognized by the ACGME as tracking and reporting faculty development will be part of the requirements effective in 2017. Faculty usually come from varying training environments and are apt to teach the way they were taught. It is useful to recognize that there is often little education for faculty as evaluators in the operating room. There is a 50-year history of a successful orthopaedic educator's course provided once a year in November by the AAOS. The ACGME frequently offers courses in resident assessment, using milestones, and other educator's skills. The Council of Orthopaedic Residency Directors provides a short half-day meeting in conjunction with the AAOS meeting in March, and a longer dedicated conference in conjunction with AOA in June. The challenges are finding time for orthopaedic educators to be away from clinical demands regardless of whether available efforts are local or provided nationally.

No single formula will work well for all training, but developing a culture of regular constructive feedback and evaluation is helpful and this starts with the residents. The experience with simulation and other hands-on observed training efforts supports the idea that residents welcome feedback as a way to progress technical skills. A global skill evaluation close to the time of evaluation can help provide specific and constructive feedback for a wide range of procedures. Task-specific scores like ASSET are under development in many areas. Widespread measurement of resident operative performance also promises to support curriculum development, identify best practices, and explore the strengths and weaknesses of our current system of orthopaedic training. Some of this will be mandated by our accreditation and assessment organizations, and some of it will come from innovation within the programs themselves.

Conclusion

Medicine evolves continuously—issues like physician burnout and mandates like milestones were not a part of life as a program director 10 years ago and yet we are now responsible for both. It is easy to feel like there is just too much concept and not enough practical reality! Perhaps this chapter hasn't helped that, but at the minimum self-education about the options provides a place to start. The challenge for our specialty moving forward is to measure, adapt, and adopt the processes that work and to be creative where we need to. Our emphasis should be on developing tools and educational structures designed to assess and inform the learner with the ultimate goal of both knowledge and technical skill improvement. Our strength is in recognizing the strengths and weaknesses of our residencies both locally and at a national level; we are not "one size fits all," but neither are we ridiculously different. The mission of orthopaedic educators today should be education done purposefully because purpose is inherent to who we are.

References

1. Bok HG, Jaarsma DA, Spruijt A, Van Beukelen P, Van Der Vleuetn CP, Teunissen PW. Feedback-giving behavior in performance evaluations during clinical clerkships. Med Teach. 2016;38(1):88–95.
2. Crossley J, Jolly B. Making sense of work-based assessment: ask the right questions, in the right way, about the right things, of the right people. Med Educ. 2012;46(1):28–37.
3. Govaerts M, van der Vleuten CP. Validity in work-based assessment: expanding our horizons. Med Educ. 2013;47(12):1164–74.
4. Rekman J, Hamstra SJ, Dudek N, Wood T, Seabrook C, Gofton W. A new instrument for assessing resident competence in surgical clinic: the Ottawa Clinic Assessment Tool. J Surg Educ. 2016;73(4):575–82.
5. Van der Vleuten C, Verhoeven B. In-training assessment developments in postgraduate education in Europe. ANZ J Surg. 2013;83(6):454–9.

6. Dudek NL, Marks MB, Regehr G. Failure to fail: the perspectives of clinical supervisors. Acad Med. 2005;80(10 Suppl):S84–7.
7. Evaniew N, Holt G, Kreuger S, Farrokhyar F, Petrisor B, Dore K, Bhandari M, Ghert M. The orthopaedic in-training examination: perspectives of program directors and residents from the United States and Canada. J Surg Educ. 2013;70(4):528–36.
8. Haughom BD, Goldstein Z, Hellman MD, Yi PH, Frank RM, Levine BR. An analysis of references used for the Orthopaedic In-Training Examination: what are their levels of evidence and journal impact factors? Clin Orthop Relat Res. 2014;472(12):4024–32.
9. LaPorte DM, Marker DR, Seyler TM, Mont MA, Frassica FJ. Educational resources for the Orthopedic In-Training Examination. J Surg Educ. 2010;67(3):135–8.
10. Krueger CA, Shakir I, Fuller BC. Prevalence of answers to orthopaedic in-training examination questions in 3 commonly used orthopedic review sources. Orthopedics. 2012;35(9):e1420–6.
11. Herndon JH, Allan BJ, Dyer G, Jawa A, Zurakowski D. Predictors of success on the American Board of Orthopaedic Surgery examination. Clin Orthop Relat Res. 2009;467(9):2436–45.
12. Dougherty PJ, Walter N, Schilling P, Najibi S, Herkowitz H. Do scores of the USMLE Step 1 and OITE correlate with the ABOS Part I certifying examination? A multicenter study. Clin Orthop Relat Res. 2010;468(10):2797–802.
13. Swanson D, Marsh JL, Hurwitz S, DeRosa GP, Holtzman K, Bucak SD, Baker A, Morrison C. Utility of AAOS OITE scores in predicting ABOS Part I outcomes: AAOS exhibit selection. J Bone Joint Surg Am. 2013;95(12):e84.
14. Ponce B, Savage J, Momaya A, Seales J, Oliver J, McGwin G, Theiss S. Association between orthopaedic in-training examination subsection scores and ABOS Part 1 examination performance. South Med J. 2014;107(12):746–50.
15. Miller GE. The assessment of clinical skills/competence/performance. Acad Med. 1990;65(9 Suppl):S63–7.
16. Pitts D, Rowley DI, Sher JL. Assessment of performance in orthopaedic training. J Bone Joint Surg Br. 2005;87(9):1187–91.
17. Schuwirth L, Colliver J, Gruppen L, Kreiter C, Mennin S, Onishi H, Pangaro L, Ringsted C, Swanson D, Van Der Vleuten C, Wagner-Menghin M. Research in assessment: consensus statement and recommendations from the Ottawa 2010 Conference. Med Teach. 2011;33(3):224–33.
18. Norcini JJ, Blank LL, Arnold GK, Kimball HR. The mini-CEX (clinical evaluation exercise): a preliminary investigation. Ann Intern Med. 1995;123(10):795–9.

19. Nair BK, Moonen-van Loon JM, Parvathy MS, van der Vleuten CP. Composite reliability of workplace-based assessment for international medical graduates. Med J Aust. 2016;205(5):212–6.
20. Lee V, Brain K, Martin J. Factors influencing mini-CEX rater judgments and their practical implications: a systematic literature review. Acad Med. 2017;92(6), 880–88.
21. Durning SJ, Cation LJ, Markert RJ, Pangaro LN. Assessing the reliability and validity of the mini-clinical evaluation exercise for internal medicine residency training. Acad Med. 2002;77(9):900–4.
22. Al Ansari A, Ali SK, Donnon T. The construct and criterion validity of the mini-CEX: a meta-analysis of the published research. Acad Med. 2013;88(3):413–20.
23. Wilson AB, Choi JN, Torbeck LJ, Mellinger JD, Dunnington GL, Williams RG. Clinical Assessment and Management Examination—Outpatient (CAMEO): its validity and use in a surgical milestones paradigm. J Surg Educ. 2015;72(1):33–40.
24. Ten Cate O, Hart D, Ankel F, Busari J, Englander R, Glasgow N, Holmboe E, Iobst W, Lovell E, Snell LS, Touchie C, Van Melle E. Wycliffe-Jones K; International Competency-Based Medical Education Collaborators. Entrustment Decision Making in Clinical Training. Acad Med. 2016;91(2):191–8.
25. Frankel RM, Eddins-Folensbee F, Inui TS. Crossing the patient-centered divide: transforming health care quality through enhanced faculty development. Acad Med. 2011;86(4):445–52.
26. Lesser CS, Lucey CR, Egener B, Braddock CH, Linas SL, Levinson W. A behavioral and systems view of professionalism. JAMA. 2010;304(24):2732–7.
27. Lundine K, Buckley R, Hutchison C, Lockyer J. Communication skills training in orthopaedics. J Bone Joint Surg Am. 2008;90(6):1393–400.
28. Tongue JR, Epps HR, Forese LL. Communication Skills. Instr Course Lect. 2005;54:3–9.
29. Davis DA, Mazmanian PE, Fordis M, Van Harrison R, Thorpe KE, Perrier L. Accuracy of physician self-assessment compared with observed measures of competence: a systematic review. JAMA. 2006;296(9):1094–102.
30. Phillips D, Zuckerman JD, Strauss EJ, Egol KA. Objective Structured Clinical Examinations: a guide to development and implementation in orthopaedic residency. J Am Acad Orthop Surg. 2013;21(10):592–600.

31. Alderson D. Developing expertise in surgery. Med Teach. 2010;32(10):830–6.
32. Winckel CP, Reznick RK, Cohen R, Taylor B. Reliability and construct validity of a structured technical skills assessment form. Am J Surg. 1994;167(4):423–7.
33. Martin JA, Regehr G, Reznick R, MacRae H, Murnaghan J, Hutchison C, Brown M. Objective structured assessment of technical skill (OSATS) for surgical residents. Br J Surg. 1997;84(2):273–8.
34. Hopmans CJ, den Hoed PT, van der Laan L, van der Harst E, van der Elst M, Mannaerts GH, Dawson I, Timman R, Wijnhoven BP, IJzermans JN. Assessment of surgery residents' operative skills in the operating theater using a modified Objective Structured Assessment of Technical Skills (OSATS): a prospective multi-center study. Surgery. 2014;156(5):1078–88.
35. Hatala R, Cook DA, Brydges R, Hawkins R. Constructing a validity argument for the Objective Structured Assessment of Technical Skills (OSATS): a systematic review of validity evidence. Adv Health Sci Educ Theory Pract. 2015;20(5):1149–75.
36. Anderson DD, Long S, Thomas GW, Putnam MD, Bechtold JE, Karam MD. Objective Structured Assessments of Technical Skills (OSATS) does not assess the quality of the surgical result effectively. Clin Orthop Relat Res. 2016;474(4):874–81.
37. Steigerwald SN, Park J, Hardy KM, Gillman L, Vergis AS. Establishing the concurrent validity of general and technique-specific skills assessments in surgical education. Am J Surg. 2016;211(1):268–73.
38. Egol KA, Phillips D, Vongbandith T, Szyld D, Strauss E. Do orthopaedic fracture skills courses improve resident performance? Injury. 2015;46(4):547–51.
39. Insel A, Carofino B, Leger R, Arciero R, Mazzocca AD. The development of an objective model to assess arthroscopic performance. J Bone Joint Surg Am. 2009;91(9):2287–95.
40. Koehler RJ, Amsdell S, Arendt EA, Bisson LJ, Braman JP, Butler A, Cosgarea AJ, Harner CD, Garrett WE, Olson T, Warme WJ, Nicandri GT. The arthroscopic surgical skill evaluation tool (ASSET). Am J Sports Med. 2013;41(6):1229–37.
41. Gofton WT, Dudek NL, Wood TJ, Balaa F, Hamstra SJ. The Ottawa surgical competency operating room evaluation (O-SCORE): a tool to assess surgical competence. Acad Med. 2012;87(10):1401–7.

42. MacEwan MJ, Dudek NL, Wood TJ, Gofton WT. Continued validation of the O-SCORE (Ottawa Surgical Competency Operating Room Evaluation): use in the simulated environment. Teach Learn Med. 2016;28(1):72–9.
43. Hopmans CJ, den Hoed PT, Wallenburg I, van der Laan L, van der Harst E, van der Elst M, Mannaerts GH, Dawson I, van Lanschot JJ, Ijzermans JN. Surgeons' attitude toward a competency-based training and assessment program: results of a multicenter survey. J Surg Educ. 2013;70(5):647–54.
44. DaRosa DA, Zwischenberger JB, Meyerson SL, George BC, Teitelbaum EN, Soper NJ, Fryer JP. A theory-based model for teaching and assessing residents in the operating room. J Surg Educ. 2013;70(1):24–30.
45. Howells NR, Brinsden MD, Gill RS, Carr AJ, Rees JL. Motion analysis: a validated method for showing skill levels in arthroscopy. Arthroscopy. 2008;24(3):335–42.
46. Tashiro Y, Miura H, Nakanishi Y, Okazaki K, Iwamoto Y. Evaluation of skills in arthroscopic training based on trajectory and force data. Clin Orthop Relat Res. 2009;467(2):546–52.

Chapter 8
Providing Feedback to Residents

Vani Sabesan and James Whaley

Introduction

Who would dispute the idea that feedback is a good thing? Both common sense and research make it clear: Formative assessment, consisting of lots of feedback and opportunities to use that feedback, enhances performance and achievement [1]. John Hattie (2008), whose decades of research revealed that feedback was among the most powerful influences on achievement, acknowledges that he has "struggled to understand the concept" [2]. Many writings on the subject don't even attempt to define the term. To improve formative assessment practices among both teachers and learners, we need to look more closely at just what feedback is—and isn't.

V. Sabesan, MD (✉)
Program Director and Associate Professor, Department of
Orthopaedic Surgery, Beaumont Health System/Wayne
State University, 18100 Oakwood Blvd. Suite 300, Dearborn,
48124 MI, USA
e-mail: sabes001@gmail.com

J. Whaley, MD
Associate Professor, Department of Orthopaedic Surgery,
Wayne State University, Cleveland Clinic, 2950 Cleveland Clinic
Boulevard, Weston, 33331 FL, USA

P.J. Dougherty, B.L. Joyce (eds.), *The Orthopedic Educator*,
DOI 10.1007/978-3-319-62944-5_8

The Accreditation Council for Graduate Medical Education (ACGME) requires residency programs to document trainee performance, and provide more continuous feedback during training. Specifically, the goal of any surgical residency is to prepare residents to not only be board-certified surgeons, but also achieve competency to become good physicians [3, 4]. Improvement in operating skills, for example, requires constant feedback between teacher and learner to promote reflection on performance [3, 4]. In the new era of milestones, effective feedback is critical in developing competent surgeons; however, studies report that feedback can be lacking [5, 6]. Orthopaedic surgery training programs utilize the apprenticeship model, based on the idea that the master teaches the trainee, and the trainee engages in experiential learning or learning by doing [7]. Resident feedback, in the apprenticeship model, is an essential part of creating competent orthopaedic surgeons. Traditionally, feedback in residency training was at the end of rotation, informal, subjective, and vague [8]. There were problems with this type of feedback in that the timeliness and quality of the evaluation were suboptimal [6, 9]. One study of orthopaedic residents at a single institution showed that almost half of residents felt that they received immediate surgical feedback less than 20% of the time [9]. Moreover, a department review of 1556 faculty evaluations of residents over 4 years showed that the average time to receive written feedback was 43 days after the rotation ended [9]. Feedback is necessary for the growth of the resident into a competent surgeon. In a time now with emphasis on milestones and competency curriculum, effective feedback is a critical component of residency training and faculty are sought out to provide high-quality feedback that encourages residents to engage in deliberate practice to refine their skills [10, 11].

What Is Feedback?

Feedback can be defined as "specific information about the comparison between trainee's observed performance and a standard given with the intent to improve trainee's performance" (p. 193) [12]. The term *feedback* is often used to describe all kinds of comments made after the fact, including advice, praise, and evaluation. But feedback is ill defined. Basically, feedback is information about how we are performing in our efforts to reach a goal. I tell a joke with the goal of making people laugh, and I observe the audience's reaction—they laugh loudly or barely snicker. I teach a lesson with the goal of engaging students, and I see that some students have their eyes riveted on me while others are nodding off. Because the term feedback may be used to describe a number of scenarios, it can often be overlooked by residents. Defined another way, feedback is the process of the resident seeking to find out more about the similarities and differences between their performance and the target performance [13, 14]. This definition emphasizes the active role of the resident, as they have to be motivated in implementing the learning plans to achieve a target performance [13–16]. Specific feedback must instruct the resident on what the target performance is and how their performance differs [13, 15, 16]. Although there is no consensus on the definition of feedback, one review found that three concepts emerged: feedback as information, feedback as reactive to information that is given, and feedback as cyclic, involving information and reaction [12]. To expand on this, feedback as information is essentially the information on the learner's performance, with the focus on content of the information. Feedback as a reaction differs, in that there is an interchange of information delivery and reception, where the focus is on the interaction with information. Lastly, feedback as a cycle is when the output is fed back as the new input to modify and improve future outputs, with the focus being on receiving information, responding to the information, and improving response quality [12].

There are many forms and avenues for feedback including formal or informal, clinical and surgical, reinforcing or corrective, and verbal or written. Ultimately, there are two main types of feedback: formative ongoing feedback which occurs on a regular or an ad hoc basis, and summative (formal) feedback which is typically shared during annual or semiannual performance reviews. Formal summative feedback usually occurs in a meeting-type environment or as a formalized document, such as an individualized learning plan. Formative feedback (informal), on the other hand, is characterized as "on the fly" and less directive. The feedback may address behavior in the operating room or the clinic, with each situation addressing different aspects of the resident's performance. All feedback is not corrective; if a resident is performing well, feedback can be given to reinforce the good behaviors and point out performance strengths. Lastly, feedback may be written or oral, with written feedback usually comprising some sort of numerical grading system that allows for tracking of residents' progress over time and also a comments section. Simple oral feedback models have been developed to allow for real-time ongoing assessments, both in the clinic and in the operating room.

Regardless of the form, the seven main components of high-quality feedback are goal referenced, tangible and transparent, actionable, user friendly, timely, ongoing, and consistent [1, 2, 5, 17]. Feedback, most importantly, should avoid disrespectful or personal comments that have a judgment or focus on the personality and not on specific behavior, not be goal oriented, and provide no constructive suggestions for improvement [18, 19].

Types of Feedback

Research has found that choosing the right types of feedback strategy and content specific to the learning target is the most important for student achievement. Definitions and examples of types of feedback are included below. It is important to remember that any feedback given must be cognizant of tone, clarity, and specificity which are critical for any type of feedback.

Written feedback: Feedback that is in the written language and is often provided in the middle and end of a rotation and is usually formal: The evaluative form usually has a component of written feedback. With the goal for residents to improve performance or address areas of weakness, short phrases of nonspecific comments are suboptimal such as "Good job" or "Hard worker." The faculty member needs to elaborate on their overall impression of the residence's performance. For instance, explain why the resident did a good job, and offer goals and plans to achieve them that are tailored to the resident's experience level. Integrate "sandwich-type" evaluation or other specific models; add examples and be specific and directive in how resident can improve.

Verbal feedback: Feedback that is spoken and should occur on a daily basis that is focused on improvement of the resident's clinical and surgical skills throughout the rotation: The majority of the time this type of feedback is informal because it takes place "on the go." When giving this type of feedback faculty need to be aware of critical components including the language used, location, identifying and defining the teachable moment, and tone. Language and tone are important because you can say the same thing, and have it interpreted differently based on whether an aggressive or a calm tone and inviting or open language were used. Confrontational tones (aggressive, condescending, and sarcastic) will put the resident into a defensive mode and they are unlikely to act on the feedback.

Formal feedback: Feedback that is provided as part of a summative assessment: The feedback is mostly written, and covers the resident's performance both clinically and surgically. There may be a verbal component if the faculty member and resident meet to go over the assessment. This type of feedback follows the resident throughout their training and allows for improvement to be seen longitudinally in the long term. An important note is that the faculty member needs to be specific and descriptive because that will allow for a more accurate measure of the resident's improvement longitudinally throughout residency.

Informal (ongoing) feedback: Feedback that takes place on a day-to-day basis with the goal of improving the resident's performance for that rotation: The feedback is usually verbal, and can occur in the clinic or operating room. When giving this feedback, the faculty member needs to help the resident set a goal for improvement and a plan to get there. For example, saying "your shoulder exam needs to be improved" is not as helpful as more specific feedback like "your shoulder exam lacked testing for impingement or strength" or "I have found that this book chapter is a great resource, please read it tonight and we will go over it tomorrow."

Feedback Models

Any good model of delivering feedback should assess orientation and climate, and include elicitation, diagnosis and feedback, improvement plan, application, and review [18]. It is best to let the resident know ahead of time that there will be a feedback session to orient them for the session, and it is the faculty member's responsibility to provide a relaxed and respectful climate [18]. This also allows the resident to manage their duties and optimizes the ability for them to be mentally engaged in the session.

To start the session off, elicit from the resident a self-assessment and use open-ended questions about the resident's performance [7, 18, 20]. This is important because it allows you, as faculty, to understand the resident's perception of their performance, to engage them in the process, and to begin to formulate a focus area for improvement. During the conversation, provide reinforcing and corrective feedback, as well as responses (diagnosis) to the observations of the resident [18]. The faculty should also use their expertise to help clarify misunderstandings, set priorities, and offer suggestions for improvement [13].

Next is to develop specific strategies for improvement, or improvement plan, by giving your suggestions, and asking the resident how they can improve [18, 21]. The most important step is the resident applying the discussed strategies to the present time and, as a faculty member, it is your job to monitor the development and application of the improvement plan [18]. Lastly, have the resident repeat back what was discussed at the session. This review allows for identification of any misinterpretations, and allows the faculty member and resident to agree on a timeline for change [18]. The goal of the session is for it to be a dialogue and constructive, not paternalistic, condescending, or insulting [13]. Having the resident engaged in his/her own strategy for improvement will lead to the resident being more likely to implement the changes, and ultimately allow them to be a better orthopaedic surgeon [13].

A simplistic model of feedback recently propagated is the One-Minute Preceptor model. This model has been used in many leadership programs, emphasized in orthopaedic surgery educational programs, utilized by faculty in graduate medical education, and provides a simple yet effective real-time model for providing feedback to residents [22, 23]. In this model the first step is getting a commitment from the resident by finding out their diagnosis or plan or how they think they did. Next, you want to probe for supporting evidence to understand why the resident developed that thought process. After that, the faculty should teach general rules by giving the resident "take-home points" aimed at the resident's area of gaps in knowledge. The fourth step is to reinforce what was done well, positive feedback, and what the resident should continue to do. Lastly, provide constructive feedback to correct any errors that you identified along with suggestions on how to improve.

Pendleton's rules are another popular conventional model for feedback [24]. The first part is the resident's self-assessment of what they did well. The faculty member then reinforces what was done well, as well as what skills were necessary to achieve the successful outcome. Next, the resident gives another self-assessment, but this time on what could have performed better. This includes analyzing the skills used that lead to these suboptimal results. The faculty member can then suggest alternative ways to achieve the target level of performance. The benefit of this approach is that strengths are discussed first, which allows for a comfortable environment to be created with a receptive resident.

Another more simplistic feedback model is the feedback sandwich [24, 25]. In the first step of this three-step process the faculty member delivers positive feedback to the resident (top layer of bread). Next, the faculty member gives constructive feedback based on the resident's performance on a certain task or task (meat of the sandwich). Lastly, the faculty member ends the sessions with more positive feedback (bottom layer of bread). This model is generally well received by the resident as the guidance for improvement is comfortable for the learner. However, the resident may take away only the positive comments provided in the encounter and dismiss the constructive criticisms. Without the resident focusing on the constructive criticism, the goal to improve performance can be missed.

Finally there is also the CAST model for delivering effective feedback to residents [26]. CAST stands for Continue, Alter, Stop, Try. Initially during the encounter, the faculty member acknowledges the behaviors that the resident should continue to do. Next, the resident is informed of behaviors that need to be altered so that they can become strengths. After that, the faculty member discusses what activities need to be stopped because they do not add value, or are applied the wrong way. Lastly, the faculty member offers new skills to apply and practice for the resident to try the next time.

Similar to the CAST model, the SKS method is a three-step feedback method that stands for Stop, Keep, Start [27]. This method is one that is usually used by the resident who seeks feedback. The first step addresses what the resident should stop doing. The second step encourages residents to keep doing certain behaviors or maintain the positives. Finally, in the third step, the faculty encourages the resident to start doing or to try a new behavior. This method allows for a very brief encounter that can be impactful. Furthermore, this is a model that can be utilized by residents to regularly seek feedback. The SKS method does rely on the resident to be self-reflective and receptive to feedback because a perceived strength may actually be viewed as a weakness by faculty.

Location of the Feedback

The one-on-one environment of the clinic is a crucial time to provide low-stakes formative assessment and constructive feedback [28]. The clinic allows the faculty member to evaluate aspects outside of the operating room, such as communication, empathy, diagnostic skills, exam skills, interpretation of imaging, and decision making and critical thinking skills. Try to avoid giving a resident feedback near the patient rooms or public areas, as this may make the resident uncomfortable and hinder an open discussion. Again, it is important to emphasize that the feedback session is a dialogue, and the resident should be actively participating in the discussion. A goal after each day of clinic is to have a brief debriefing meeting with the resident, and address goals set and previous plans for improvement, if those goals have been achieved, modifying previous plans for improvement, and creation of new plans of improvement. The easiest way to implement the short debriefing processes is to do it after the last patient is seen; this takes a maximum of 5 min. Focusing on one area of improvement allows for the session to be brief, effective, and allow everyone to finish their clinic work.

Surgical feedback provides residents with ways to improve their operative skills. Delivering this information can prove to be difficult due to the fast-paced environment of the operating room, but is critical for development. Feedback needs to be frequent and temporally close to when a procedure was performed. An immediate brief postoperative debriefing has been shown to be effective with minimal time used [20]. The impact of feedback can be powerful in the surgical setting by allowing the resident to obtain surgical skills at higher level of proficiency or even faster [29]. The One-Minute Preceptor model previously described can be utilized effectively in between surgical cases, given the time constraints that can be associated with the operating room. The feedback can range anywhere from preoperative preparation to surgical technique and intraoperative performance.

A great way to provide surgical skill feedback is during simulation labs, such as a cadaveric lab or a sawbones lab. This is a low-stress environment that allows for feedback to be instantaneous during a procedure, and allows for the resident to make corrections in real time. In addition, the clearer the expectations are set for performance the more fruitful feedback can be after a case for a resident.

Tips for Providing Residents with Meaningful Feedback

There are similarities and differences in feedback in the clinic and in the operating room. Both arenas are valuable times to provide meaningful feedback that will help improve residence performance. Furthermore, both situations require the faculty member to give feedback that is goal oriented, tangible, actionable, resident friendly, timely, ongoing, and consistent [1, 2, 5, 17]. Admittedly, the operating room is a more high-stress environment than the clinic, and it is important to avoid disrespectful or personal comments that focus on the resident's personality [18, 19]. The operating room is a crucial component of orthopaedic surgical training as it allows the resident to perform under the direct supervision of the attending [30]. Feedback in the operating room is provided in real time and directed at improving procedural performance of the resident, as well as maintaining patient safety. Additionally, improvement can be rapid and, therefore, the faculty member must continue to provide feedback until the target performance is achieved. This immediate feedback is vital, as waiting until the end of the rotation to give feedback is suboptimal because of selective recall and errors due to forgetting [31, 32]. The goal of feedback in the operating room is to develop an efficient, skilled, independent, and autonomous surgeon [33].

Five Important Tips

1. Create safety: If the resident doesn't feel comfortable, then the feedback will be unproductive. Making the resident feel bad or embarrassing them in front of their peers is not productive.
2. Be positive: Being positive allows the resident to feel comfortable and make them more likely to actively participate in the conversation. Even if corrective feedback is needed, follow that up with a solution or an achievable goal.
3. Be specific: Specific observations of behavior allow the resident to focus on what exactly needs to be addressed, and what steps need to be taken for improvement. Ambiguity leads to interpretation, and may lead to the resident missing the point of the feedback.
4. Be immediate: Giving feedback after a surgical case or a patient presentation allows the situation to be fresh in the faculty and resident's mind, and allows for a more accurate assessment of performance.
5. Be tough, not mean: Ask the resident their perspective and then stay objective, and address the behavior and not criticize them personally.

Optimal Feedback Model (Authors' Preferred Model)

One-Minute Preceptor Model

The author prefers this model for giving feedback on a daily basis. This model is not only providing the resident feedback on performance but also has an educational component. The One-Minute Preceptor model encourages the resident to articulate their diagnostic reasoning so they do not rely on faculty to provide the diagnosis or treatment methodology.

This model can be effectively implemented in the operating room and the clinic because of the minimal time requirement needed for an impactful resident interaction. The author encourages faculty to have different models in their repertoire, and to adapt the models to the faculty member's own style.

Pitfalls and Perils

Feedback is a multifactorial complex and is affected by learning culture, relationships, purpose of feedback, and emotional response to feedback [34]. Residents may feel that the faculty member may be unapproachable, and therefore will not seek out feedback [35]. The faculty member may not take the time to give feedback or be reluctant to give feedback because they may not have confidence in their feedback skills, or do not want to be perceived as mean or damage the relationship with the resident [13, 18, 19, 35–38]. The feedback plan may not always be implemented if the resident perceives that there is not a problem, the feedback is irrelevant, or the source is not credible [39–42]. This is especially true if the resident has a negative emotional response to the feedback [41].

There is often a difference in perception of feedback between residents and faculty members. Specifically, residents and faculty members do not share the same understanding of when feedback is being given or perception of the quality and frequency of feedback, with the residents viewing the quality and frequency as lower [3, 33, 43]. To further this point, one study of surgery residents and faculty found significant difference on how feedback was received (starting with a positive, resident participation, concrete suggestions for improvement) and how it was given (frequency and timeliness) [43]. For example, they found that 96.6% of surgeons believed that they started with a positive observation, and allowed the resident to participate in the discussion 97% of the time, and 96.4% felt that they gave concrete suggestions for improvement; the residents disagreed (54.2%, 50%, and 13%, respectively) [43]. Additionally, 86.2% of surgeons felt that they gave feedback often and always immediately after the activity, whereas 12.5% of residents felt this to be true [43]. Written feedback has been found to be short and nonspecific, which is of little value to residents seeking to improve their skills [5, 21]. Examples would include "needs to read more" or "needs improvement on physical exam" are not specific enough for the resident to use the comments effectively. However, one study showed that there is no difference between verbal or written feedback in terms of effectiveness, but rather the frequency or timeliness is a more important factor [44]. Making time for feedback can be difficult, for multiple reasons, including different resident and faculty member work schedules and duties [35]. Although faculty members' time is constrained with clinical and personal duties, it is important to take the time to craft thoughtful and high-quality feedback.

Feedback to Different Types of Residents

The Underperformer [45]

Regardless of the metrics that used for resident selection, there are always those residents who will be underperforming, even after feedback to help them improve. For some, it is due to a lack of trying, while for others orthopaedics might just not be the right fit. Regardless of the cause, the faculty need to take action as soon as possible. The most disadvantageous thing a faculty member can do is to assume that the inadequate performance will self-correct. When providing feedback to this resident it is important to engage the resident in the feedback process, state objectively what you are observing, set goals for improvement, and create an improvement plan together. The faculty can even go as far as having the resident write down agreed-upon goals and deadlines for these goals. However, some residents may not be coachable or not want to change, which leads us to our next type of resident: the defensive resident.

The Defensive Resident [45]

Difficult residents are, in the author's opinion, the most difficult resident to work with. These residents do not do well with feedback for a few reasons. They may not realize that there is a problem, and feel that the faculty member is personally attacking them, or not think that the feedback is credible, or become defensive and not accept personal responsibility. This type of resident may "twist your words," and become emotional quickly. Although this is a difficult situation to be in when delivering feedback, there are a few tips to help the resident understand the problem, and be receptive for improvement. First, the faculty member must be clear with what they say so that the resident understands fully what is being addressed. If the resident begins to twist what you are saying, simply repeat back what you said. As the faculty member, it is important to keep a neutral tone to minimize escalating the emotions of the resident. Tone is the body language, facial expressions, and voice inflection that accompany your verbal message. This is probably the hardest part about dealing with a defensive resident because it is easy for the emotions of the faculty to be shown through. Lastly, feedback should use temperate phrasing because a certain phrasing can evoke an emotional response more than others. For example, saying "You are terrible at suturing!" evokes a stronger emotional response than saying "Your suture technique needs to be improved." with the resident being more receptive to the latter phrasing. This can be accomplished by explaining how you came to your observation, asking for the resident's reaction to your feedback, and asking their perspective. Remember that your job is to give objective feedback in a clear, neutral, and temperate way.

The Star Performer [45]

In orthopaedic residency training, this type of resident can be surprisingly difficult to give feedback to. These residents are self-driven and well read, and have tirelessly practiced their surgical skills. For faculty members, it may seem difficult to find an area that is lacking, or you may feel as though you are being too critical. An important note is that your resident will be receptive to your feedback because they did not become a top performer without self-improvement. One way to approach the resident is to ask them about their goals and find out what barriers they feel are present. At this point, the faculty member may use different approaches to provide feedback to help accomplish the resident's goals. Do not be afraid to give the resident constructive feedback. An example would be saying, "Your performance is above your training level; however, I think there needs improvement in communication in the operating room." The resident may be surprised at first because they are not used to receiving constructive feedback, but they will usually use the feedback to improve.

Conclusion

Providing effective resident feedback can be very challenging for orthopaedic faculty members. Residents are eager for feedback because they believe that it can help them improve their skills [18, 46].

High-quality feedback is specific, frequent, timely, interactive, and behavioral rather than personal, and provides a plan to improve performance [5, 17]. Tailoring the above feedback models to your own personal style allows for an interactive and conversational session. This resident-centered approach allows for high-quality feedback to be provided in an effective model that will allow resident to grow into a competent and successful orthopaedic surgeon.

References

1. Wiggins G. Seven keys to effective feedback. Educ Leadersh. 2012;70(1):10–6.
2. Hattie J. Visible learning a synthesis of over 800 meta-analyses relating to achievement. Hoboken: Taylor & Francis; 2008.

3. Jensen AR, Wright AS, Kim S, Horvath KD, Calhoun KE. Educational feedback in the operating room: a gap between resident and faculty perceptions. Am J Surg. 2012;204(2):248–55.
4. Jeray KJ, Frick SL. A survey of resident perspectives on surgical case minimums and the impact on milestones, graduation, credentialing, and preparation for practice: AOA critical issues. J Bone Joint Surg Am. 2014;96(23):e195.
5. Jackson JL, Kay C, Jackson WC, Frank M. The quality of written feedback by attendings of internal medicine residents. J Gen Intern Med. 2015;30(7):973–8.
6. Weinstein DF. Feedback in clinical education: untying the Gordian knot. Acad Med. 2015;90(5):559–61.
7. Connolly A, Hansen D, Schuler K, Galvin SL, Wolfe H. Immediate surgical skills feedback in the operating room using "SurF" cards. J Grad Med Educ. 2014;6(4):774–8.
8. Angus S, Moriarty J, Nardino RJ, Chmielewski A, Rosenblum MJ. Internal medicine residents' perspectives on receiving feedback in milestone format. J Grad Med Educ. 2015;7(2):220–4.
9. Gundle KR, Mickelson DT, Hanel DP. Reflections in a time of transition: orthopaedic faculty and resident understanding of accreditation schemes and opinions on surgical skills feedback. Med Educ Online. 2016;21:30584.
10. Karam MD, Thomas GW, Koehler DM, Westerlind BO, Lafferty PM, Ohrt GT, et al. Surgical coaching from head-mounted video in the training of fluoroscopically guided articular fracture surgery. J Bone Joint Surg Am. 2015;97(12):1031–9.
11. Karam MD, Westerlind B, Anderson DD, Marsh JL. Development of an orthopaedic surgical skills curriculum for post-graduate year one resident learners - the University of Iowa experience. Iowa Orthop J. 2013;33:178–84.
12. van de Ridder JM, Stokking KM, McGaghie WC, ten Cate OT. What is feedback in clinical education? Med Educ. 2008;42(2):189–97.
13. Johnson CE, Keating JL, Boud DJ, Dalton M, Kiegaldie D, Hay M, et al. Identifying educator behaviours for high quality verbal feedback in health professions education: literature review and expert refinement. BMC Med Educ. 2016;16:96.
14. Hattie J, Timperley H. The power of feedback. Rev Educ Res. 2007;77(1):81–112.
15. Boud D, Molloy E, editors. What is the problem with feedback? In: Feedback in higher and professional education. London: Routledge; 2013.

16. Boud D, Molloy E, editors. Changing conceptions of feedback. In: Feedback in higher and professional education. London: Routledge; 2013. p. 11–33.
17. Skeff KM, Stratos GA, Berman J, Bergen MR. Improving clinical teaching. Evaluation of a national dissemination program. Arch Intern Med. 1992;152(6):1156–61.
18. Hewson MG, Little ML. Giving feedback in medical education: verification of recommended techniques. J Gen Intern Med. 1998;13(2):111–6.
19. Ende J. Feedback in clinical medical education. JAMA. 1983;250(6):777–81.
20. Cook MR, Watters JM, Barton JS, Kamin C, Brown SN, Deveney KE, et al. A flexible postoperative debriefing process can effectively provide formative resident feedback. J Am Coll Surg. 2015;220(5):959–67.
21. Berbano EP, Browning R, Pangaro L, Jackson JL. The impact of the Stanford Faculty Development Program on ambulatory teaching behavior. J Gen Intern Med. 2006;21(5):430–4.
22. Furney SL, Orsini AN, Orsetti KE, Stern DT, Gruppen LD, Irby DM. Teaching the one-minute preceptor: a randomized controlled trial. J Gen Intern Med. 2001;16(9):620–4.
23. Neher JO, Gordon KC, Meyer B, Stevens N. A five-step "microskills" model of clinical teaching. J Am Board Fam Pract. 1992;5(4):419–24.
24. Chowdhury RR, Kalu G. Learning to give feedback in medical education. Obstet Gynaecol. 2004;6(4):243–7.
25. LeBaron SW, Jernick J. Evaluation as a dynamic process. Fam Med. 2000;32(1):13–4.
26. Sefcik D, Petsche E. The CAST model: enhancing medical student and resident clinical performance through feedback. J Am Osteopath Assoc. 2015;115(4):196–8.
27. DeLong TJ, DeLong S. The paradox of excellence. Harv Bus Rev. 2011;89(6):119–23. 39
28. Rekman J, Hamstra SJ, Dudek N, Wood T, Seabrook C, Gofton W. A new instrument for assessing resident competence in surgical clinic: The Ottawa Clinic Assessment Tool. J Surg Educ. 2016;73(4):575–82.
29. Trehan A, Barnett-Vanes A, Carty MJ, McCulloch P, Maruthappu M. The impact of feedback of intraoperative technical performance in surgery: a systematic review. BMJ Open. 2015;5(6):e006759.

30. Chen XP, Williams RG, Sanfey HA, Smink DS. A taxonomy of surgeons' guiding behaviors in the operating room. Am J Surg. 2015;209(1):15–20.
31. Williams RG, Chen XP, Sanfey H, Markwell SJ, Mellinger JD, Dunnington GL. The measured effect of delay in completing operative performance ratings on clarity and detail of ratings assigned. J Surg Educ. 2014;71(6):e132–8.
32. Williams RG, Verhulst S, Colliver JA, Sanfey H, Chen X, Dunnington GL. A template for reliable assessment of resident operative performance: assessment intervals, numbers of cases and raters. Surgery. 2012;152(4):517–24. discussion 24-7
33. Chen XP, Williams RG, Smink DS. Do residents receive the same OR guidance as surgeons report? Difference between residents' and surgeons' perceptions of OR guidance. J Surg Educ. 2014;71(6):e79–82.
34. Delva D, Sargeant J, Miller S, Holland J, Alexiadis Brown P, Leblanc C, et al. Encouraging residents to seek feedback. Med Teach. 2013;35(12):e1625–31.
35. Reddy ST, Zegarek MH, Fromme HB, Ryan MS, Schumann SA, Harris IB. Barriers and facilitators to effective feedback: a qualitative analysis of data from multispecialty resident focus groups. J Grad Med Educ. 2015;7(2):214–9.
36. Blatt B, Confessore S, Kallenberg G, Greenberg L. Verbal interaction analysis: viewing feedback through a different lens. Teach Learn Med. 2008;20(4):329–33.
37. Kogan JR, Conforti LN, Bernabeo EC, Durning SJ, Hauer KE, Holmboe ES. Faculty staff perceptions of feedback to residents after direct observation of clinical skills. Med Educ. 2012;46(2):201–15.
38. Ende J, Pomerantz A, Erickson F. Preceptors' strategies for correcting residents in an ambulatory care medicine setting: a qualitative analysis. Acad Med. 1995;70(3):224–9.
39. Bing-You RG, Paterson J, Levine MA. Feedback falling on deaf ears: residents' receptivity to feedback tempered by sender credibility. Med Teach. 1997;19(1):40–4.
40. Lockyer J, Violato C, Fidler H. Likelihood of change: a study assessing surgeon use of multisource feedback data. Teach Learn Med. 2003;15(3):168–74.
41. Sargeant J, Mann K, Ferrier S. Exploring family physicians' reactions to multisource feedback: perceptions of credibility and usefulness. Med Educ. 2005;39(5):497–504.

42. Veloski J, Boex JR, Grasberger MJ, Evans A, Wolfson DB. Systematic review of the literature on assessment, feedback and physicians' clinical performance: BEME Guide No. 7. Med Teach. 2006;28(2):117–28.
43. Sender Liberman A, Liberman M, Steinert Y, McLeod P, Meterissian S. Surgery residents and attending surgeons have different perceptions of feedback. Med Teach. 2005;27(5):470–2.
44. Elnicki DM, Layne RD, Ogden PE, Morris DK. Oral versus written feedback in medical clinic. J Gen Intern Med. 1998;13(3):155–8.
45. HBR guide to delivering effective feedback. Boston: Harvard Business Review Press; 2016. p. 153–79.
46. Weller J, Jones A, Merry A, Jolly B, Saunders D. Investigation of trainee and specialist reactions to the mini-clinical evaluation exercise in anaesthesia: implications for implementation. Br J Anaesth. 2009;103(4):524–30.

Chapter 9
Resident Remediation and Due Process

Craig S. Roberts

Resident Remediation and Due Process

Remediation and due process are tools for the Program Director (PD) to apply to problems of unprofessional behavior and/or poor academic performance. Although the concept of due process for orthopaedic surgeons conjures up visions of courtrooms and legal arguments, the term "due process" for the purposes of this chapter is a nonlegal definition in an academic setting involving student rights [1]. This chapter discusses concepts of remediation and due process in the academic environment, reviews their application to orthopaedic surgery residency training programs, and presents a working framework for applying these concepts to unprofessional behavior and/or poor academic performance by orthopaedic residents in training.

C.S. Roberts, MD, MBA
Department of Orthopaedic Surgery Academic Office,
University of Louisville School of Medicine,
550 S. Jackson Street, 1st Floor, ACB, Louisville, KY 40292, USA
e-mail: craig.roberts@louisville.edu

© Springer International Publishing AG 2018
P.J. Dougherty, B.L. Joyce (eds.), *The Orthopedic Educator*,
DOI 10.1007/978-3-319-62944-5_9

Remediation

Remediation is "the act or process of remedying something that is undesirable or deficient" or "the act or process of providing remedial education" [2]. Dougherty and Marcus stated that "a remediation program must be available for residents who perform below expectations" [3]. Arnold stated that remediation has an important role in the professionalism of learners and faculty in orthopaedic surgery [4]. There are many models for remediation and include due process, a warning period, and confrontation to initiate remediation of the physician who has acted unprofessionally [4]. Cognitive behavioral therapy, motivational interviewing, and continuous monitoring are effective remediation techniques [4]. She also stated that remediation can appear to be intrusive, can disrupt workflow, and requires resources [4]. Resources include faculty time and expertise, educational materials, administrative support, and psychological counseling services.

Arnold also suggested that the remediation program itself has to fit the offense [4]. To evaluate a lapse in behavior one must (1) consider how clearly the behavior violates the standard of practice of medicine and the community; (2) how serious the offense is as a matter of actual or potential harm that may occur; and (3) whether the violation is intrinsically wrong [4, 5].

Arnold described an analogy between remediation and recovery from chemical dependency. Better results of remediation and rehabilitation from chemical dependency are reported in individuals that embrace professionalism in the first place, as well as those that express remorse, guilt, or empathy for those who may have been harmed. However, she noted that success rates vary tremendously [4].

Remediation is usually focused on improving behavior or performance that puts a resident, student, or faculty outside the normal range of performance, effectively making the individual an outlier. Phelan et al. in 1993 stated that "identifying and tracking students with difficulties" created an opportunity for intervention and remediation [6]. These authors were focusing on the evaluation of the noncognitive professional traits (i.e., professionalism, communication skills, teamwork) of medical students, and noted that this program can "complement systems that evaluated academic performance" [6]. Although this may not be obvious to us now, in a world where core competencies are now common parlance in medical school and residency training programs, these authors appear to have been clairvoyant.

Phelan et al. also emphasized early detection of "potential problem behavior" amenable to remediation [6]. They established a task force "to develop a system that allowed trending of potential problem behavior over several clerkships or teaching blocks while protecting both the student and the evaluator" [6]. Multiple evaluations were performed by an undergraduate medical education dean and a student progress committee [6].

In the case of a problem student, several steps took place: the student was informed about "the perceived problem, the situation discussed, and a mutually agreed upon remediation program was arranged." Interestingly, the authors termed this process mediation. In addition, these authors stated that if the "counseling and planned remediation program failed to work," the student progress committee would be informed [6]. This example of a remediation program emphasized helping the student, not penalizing them [6]. Furthermore, "only if the student failed the remediation program was the institution's academic disciplinary procedure implemented and documented in the academic record" [6]. Lastly, these authors indicated that earlier identification of student problems made it easier to develop a remediation program targeted toward a student's areas of weakness, and monitor a student's improvement [6]. Remediation programs for orthopaedic surgery residents are not well defined to my knowledge, and may be an opportunity for PDs to collaborate and share best practices. We have, in our department, used the process for remediation that is outlined (Fig. 9.1). In general, remediation should precede due process in order to demonstrate that

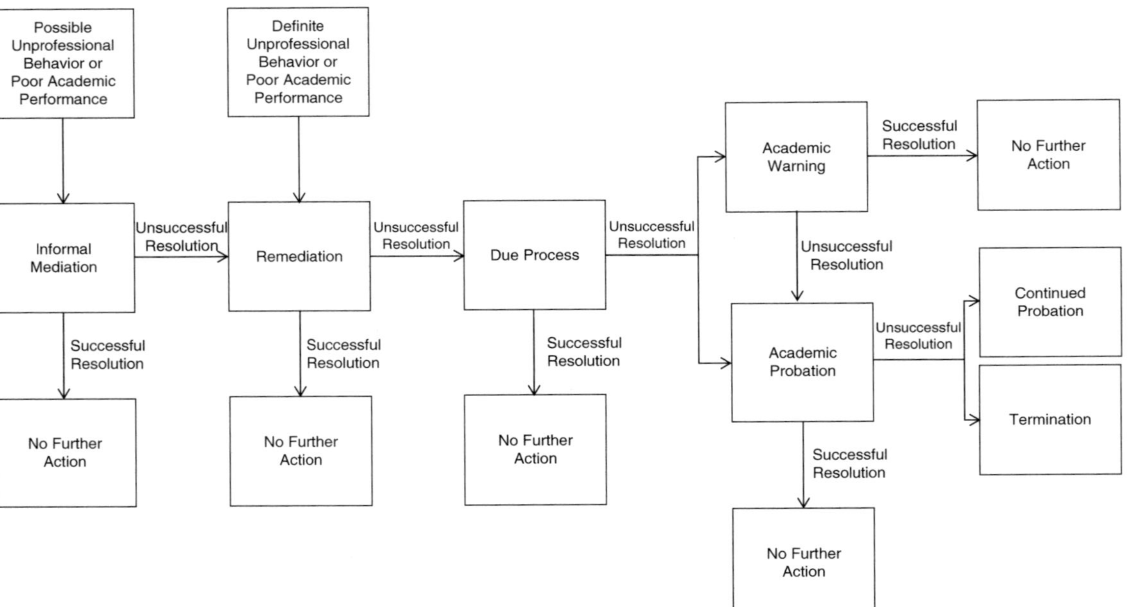

FIGURE 9.1 Working framework for applying remediation and due process to unprofessional behavior and/or poor academic performance

every effort has been made to assist the student or resident physician in improving their performance gaps.

Due Process

The *Program Directors' Handbook* notes that the "spirit of academic due process at universities involves a step-by-step process, with multiple inputs, written warnings, opportunities and resources for resident remediation, and resident retention whenever possible" [7]. This chapter further applies due process in this context.

Due process in academia is especially relevant when there is a student grievance. It ensures that the rights of the student are protected and that the individual can challenge the entire process and/or use the grievance process if desired. Most universities have grievance committees, ombudsmen, and other pathways and people to contact for these complicated situations.

In orthopaedics, PDs use the concept of due process when they are concerned that the resident's unprofessional behavior or academic performance is serious and could result in termination. Before any action in these situations, the PD ought to consult the departmental Resident Handbook, essentially the "Constitution" for educational activities [7].

How is "due process" defined in the legal arena? The concept of due process in law is associated with the Fourteenth Amendment to the Constitution of the United States where the concept of "due process of law" is imbedded [8]. In context, "No state shall … deprive any person of life, liberty, or property, without due process of law" [8].

Student rights are also mentioned discussed in the legal definition of due process. The school or institution that the student attends has written rules and policies outlining the due process procedures both students and the institution must follow to make sure that a student has a fair hearing. The idea of due process is that "no one should be assumed to have violated any laws, regulations, or ethical codes without first having a fair hearing in front of people who can judge him or her impartially, according to objective procedures, and without prejudice" [1]. The Supreme Court in 1974 heard the case of Bass VS. Lopez, a case involving students suspended without a hearing, and ruled that students have a right to due process in school [1].

Tulgan et al. discussed the development of termination policies for disruptive residents. These authors reported on their strong policies which withstood a legal challenge, and noted that strong policies are the "ultimate legal protection" [9]. Courts have generally sided with educational institutions when policies are in place and followed. Interestingly, Tulgan et al. noted that guarantees of due process for both a resident and his/her institution included the following: an unbiased tribunal; notice of the proposed action and grounds for it; opportunity to present reasons why the proposed action should not be taken; the right to present evidence, including the right to call witnesses, the right to know opposing evidence, the right to cross-examine adverse witnesses, and the right that the evidence be based exclusively on the evidence presented; and the requirement that the tribunal prepare written findings of fact and reason for its decision dependent on severity [9]. Most departments of orthopaedic surgery have all of these elements included in their policies and procedures handbook for orthopaedic residents.

A Rational Approach to Remediation and Due Process in Orthopaedic Surgery

The most common problems for the PD are the resident with a professional behavior problem or poor academic performance. There is a spectrum of problems that residents can have, from "simple and specific on one end of the spectrum, to global and complex on the other" [7]. An isolated low OITE score might require assigning a faculty mentor and a personalized study program. More global educational deficiencies (low OITE score, poor rotation evaluations, failure to progress in psychomotor skill milestones, etc.) would likely involve, at a minimum, educational mentoring and remediation by multiple faculty, prescribed review materials with standardized exams (e.g., AAOS ResStudy, Orthobullets), and psychomotor skill remediation sessions with faculty members in our arthroscopy/soft tissue skill laboratory. Determining the underlying cause of a resident's problem(s) is critical in order to be able to choose the appropriate remediation approach. The possibility of substance abuse and psychological/psychiatric issues should be considered early on, and the individual might need to be referred for the appropriate screening for substance abuse and psychological/psychiatric issues.

An initial meeting between the problem resident and the PD is a recommended first step [7]. By that point, the PD has usually received written or verbal input from others (e.g., faculty members, other residents, mid-level providers, other departments). The PD is acting almost as the third party (like a "mediator") by mediating issues or concerns among the parties involved. The PD needs to decide quickly on the scope and magnitude of the resident's problem(s), and whether it is best to start with mediation, remediation, or due process. Generally, one must not jump to due process unless there are issues of safety and immediate danger.

Although we have not discussed the details of mediation in this chapter, mediation is an informal approach and first step which is useful early on (Fig. 9.1). Mediation involves an initial conversation with the resident using active listening, a nonjudgmental approach, and careful planning for future steps so appropriate plans are in place and documentation is obtained. The PD needs to determine at the start whether the situation at hand is a problem or whether it is a dilemma. Problems, by definition, can be fixed and solved completely. Dilemmas cannot be solved, and can only be managed, generally by trade-offs and process improvement.

If the matter at hand is a simple "problem" (and not a dilemma), mediation is a good option. Mediation here is used loosely as a way or process of resolving a problem or dispute between the resident and another party, with the PD acting as a "mediator" by facilitating communication and negotiation. Academic issues such as a one-time isolated low OITE score can often be solved by the PD simply by implementing a learning/review plan or a mentoring program. Tools for mediation include informal conversations, Socratic dialogues, suggestions about modifying behavior, supplying educational resources, assigning a colleague as a study partner or accountability partner, and mentoring/coaching. Detailed documentation of this meeting is usually not critical and can be done in fairly general terms. The note of record is really a process note which records the meeting fairly succinctly [7]. This note includes the usual "who, when, what information was told or shared with you, and any action that you promised" [10]. I recommend sending the individual a letter to confirm the meeting occurred and outline what was said [7]. Copies of these notes and letters ought to be maintained for as long as possible, and will be needed for credentialing and certification for years to come [7]. Determining whether "mediation" is the correct approach is not easy, and often requires the benefit of experience. Situations which are usually not appropriate for mediation include long-standing and deep-rooted problems, people who are highly volatile, large power differences (e.g., student complains about a star faculty member), and allegations involving sexual relationship and/or those which, if proven to be true, are possibly criminal [10]. Other situations which are usually not appropriate for mediation include possible chemical dependency and substance abuse. Other options ought to be considered in these situations include referral to physician health/substance abuse programs, similar to the one in Kentucky, which are state run. In many cases with medical students and resident physicians at academic medical centers, such issues are handled internally at a departmental and/or graduate medical education level, and hospital chief medical officers are usually not involved.

The next step in the continuum of options is remediation (Fig. 9.1). Remediation can be used when simple mediation has not worked or when a defined area of unprofessional behavior or an area of difficulty, or when a gap in knowledge or performance, is identified, and is thought to be well defined and completely remediable. Some examples include poor performance on a standardized test, such as the orthopaedic in-training examination, specific knowledge gaps identified from a rotation in a particular area of orthopaedics, a behavioral skill or problem such as interaction with nursing staff in the hospital emergency room, or poor technical skills/surgical competency for a specific procedure. In these instances, an initial meeting is important to define the area which needs to be improved, identify the gap between current performance and the required performance, develop a strategy/plan on how to get there, and define what will happen if the individual does not reach the required level of performance. Documentation is more important than it is with mediation. Nonetheless, the situation has not risen to the level of due process, where the documentation is perhaps just as important as the process itself.

With remediation, documentation includes the usual "who, when, and what," and any action that you promised, in addition to describing what level of performance ("goal") has to be reached, and what will occur if this is not reached. These goals are usually accepted levels of performance, often now defined in orthopaedic residency training by the 41 ACGME orthopaedic surgery milestones. PDs should check to make sure that their resident handbook has policies and procedures for remediation and due process that align with the overall institutional GME policy and procedure manual. Definitions of professionalism and what constitutes professional behavior should align at the program level and the institutional level. When due process is required, the situation is quite serious, and the individual is at risk of future termination from the program. Although Gunsalus stated that "it is never your job to be a lawyer," due process problems and issues have considerable legal risk and are not the time to improvise [10]. Legal counsel should always be obtained early on and then periodically, as needed. For Program

Directors, a reasonable working approach to due process is to understand the policies and procedures that are already in place for the specific academic issue. Resident handbooks, which should be updated on a regular basis, are commonly distributed at the beginning of the academic year. Specific steps of disciplinary actions such as "academic warning," "academic probation," and "dismissal" are required and contained in these handbooks (Fig. 9.1). These terms should be discussed at resident orientation to familiarize every resident with what is contained in the handbook.

Sudden action without a period of time following these processes is generally unwise. Terminating a resident without progressive, stepwise discipline is usually inconsistent with the spirit of due process. However, the one exception for proceeding with immediate action such as termination is when there are issues of safety and immediate danger, in which case immediate action can be justified but will, nevertheless, be subject to scrutiny, review, legal challenge, and possible reversal at a later date. Otherwise, terminating a resident without due process is not recommended.

When an academic warning is appropriate, it is recommended that it is delivered both face to face and in writing. Academic warning should include areas of noncompliance with the departmental policies and procedures; actions and processes that need to take place to correct these areas of noncompliance; the length of the warning period; how the resident will be evaluated at the end of the period; and what might occur if the resident's behavior is unsatisfactory at the end of that period [7]. The PD also needs to do his/her homework in advance by getting inputs from others such as the Department Chair, Education Committee, and faculty [7]. The Program Director's recommendation for an action such as "probation" often has to be signed off by the Designated Institutional Officer, and may also require co-signature by the Dean of the School of Medicine. Any probationary periods must be defined in terms of duration, a precise reason, a definitive plan that outlines areas for the resident's improvement, identification of faculty/mentor responsibilities, and how performance will be assessed [7]. For example, the statement, "He did not demonstrate the knowledge, skills, and professionalism becoming of a PGY-3 resident in orthopaedic surgery." would likely be supported by unsatisfactory clinical evaluations, unsatisfactory evaluation of clinical skills, and multiple documented instances of unprofessional behavior, and possible unsatisfactory performance of written tests. Documentation is extremely important if a resident is going to be placed on probation.

The resident should always be informed of his/her rights at every step, including his/her right to contact the institutional student grievance officer/ombudsman, and the right to initiate a grievance. Lastly, the Program Director should expect that if a grievance is filed or if "dismissal" was the issue, this might be a prelude to litigation in the future.

If a resident's contract is not going to be renewed, it is important that the PD has followed due process, with the progressive steps of remediation, academic warning, and academic probation. Ideally, the possibility of a nonrenewal of the annual resident contract would have been mentioned and documented as a possible outcome if the gap or deficiency in professional behavior and/or academic performance could not be satisfactorily remediated. Also, legal counsel should be obtained well in advance by the PD if a possible nonrenewal of an annual contract is being considered.

Conclusion

There are a broad range of options available to the PD when presented with a resident with unprofessional behavior or poor academic behavior. The PD should consult legal counsel and institutional graduate medical education leadership with situations requiring due process.

Remediation and due process are essential elements of the toolbox of PDs in orthopaedic surgery. The rationale and compassionate application of remediation and due process in orthopaedic surgery require emotional intelligence and experience.

References

1. ACLU: American Civil Liberties Union of Vermont. https://acluvt.org/pubs/students_rights/due_process.php. Accessed 8/12/16.
2. American Heritage Dictionary of the English Language, 5th Edition, 2011. www.thefreedictionary.com/remediation. Accessed 8/12/2016.
3. Dougherty P, Marcus RE. ACGME and ABOS changes for the orthopaedic surgery PGY-1 (Intern) year. Clin Orthop Relat Res. 2013;471(11):3412–6.
4. Arnold L. Responding to the professionalism of learners and Faculty in Orthopaedic Surgery. Clin Orthop Relat Res. 2006;449:205–13.
5. Morrein EH. Am I my brother's warden? Responding to the unethical or incompetent colleague. Hastin Cent Rep. 1993;23:19–27.
6. Phelan S, Obenshain SS, Galey WR. Evaluation of the non-cognitive professional traits of medical students. Acad Med. 1993;68(10):799–803.
7. Roberts CS. (2013) Dealing with problems. In: Meyer FN, editor. Program director's handbook. https://issuu.com/american-orthopaedicassoc/docs/program_director_s_handbook. Accessed on 8/29/2016.
8. Cornell University Law School, Legal Information Institute, US Constitution, Amendment Fourteen, Section 1. https://www.law.cornell.edu/constitution/amendmentxiv. Accessed on 8/17/2016
9. Tulgan H, Cohen SN, Kinne KM. How a teaching hospital implemented its termination policies for disruptive residents. Acad Med. 2001;76(11):1107–12.
10. Gunsalus CK. The college administrator's survival guide. Cambridge: Hrvard Univesity Press; 2006.

Chapter 10
Faculty Development

Matthew D. Karam and J. Lawrence Marsh

Background

The mission statements of most orthopedic departments in the country that train residents place value on the delivery of excellent patient care, education of young physicians, and discovery of new medical knowledge. Traditionally academic medical centers and orthopedic departments had relatively few full-time faculty members. Their clinical commitments were less rigorous than present day's, and they were able to be more committed to the education of medical students and residents [1].

In the traditional apprenticeship model of surgical education, which has been in place for over a century, residents participate in practices of faculty members, and were allowed enough autonomy to gain experience and skills in surgical care. Residency programs were often associated with hospitals where there were less supervised environments that enhanced graduated responsibility for residents. Current surgical faculty are under pressures that have strained the traditional apprenticeship model of surgical education. These

M.D. Karam, MD (✉) • J.L. Marsh, MD
The Department of Orthopedics and Rehabilitation,
The University of Iowa Hospitals and Clinics, 200 Hawkins Drive,
Iowa City, 52242 IA, USA
e-mail: Matthew-karam@uiowa.edu; j-marsh@uiowa.edu

© Springer International Publishing AG 2018   167
P.J. Dougherty, B.L. Joyce (eds.), *The Orthopedic Educator*,
DOI 10.1007/978-3-319-62944-5_10

include pressures to bill and see more patients, emphasis on patient safety and quality, increased role of mid-level providers, and loss of resident experiences in less supervised hospital environments. Faculty must now make extra time and effort to be educators. It no longer can be just part of the system of patient care.

Young academic faculty members take on many responsibilities and roles that are in addition to learning the craft of a surgeon and the skills that are required. They work in a large enterprise with little control. They may engage in research and national organizations and committee work and aspire to positions in leadership. Being an educator is only one of these roles and education is under particular stress. The question then becomes how do programs and department leaders insure that faculty members are equipped to meet the educational needs of present-day medical students and orthopedic surgery residents and fellows, and develop the skills necessary to be good educators. With this background it is clear that development of faculty skills, aptitudes, and desire for successful engagement in the education of residents and students has become increasingly important.

Learning to Be a Surgical Educator

Effective orthopedic educators are essential to produce the top-notch orthopedic surgeons of tomorrow. Studies have highlighted the attributes of a good medical educator. Interestingly enough these attributes remain the same across all medical specialties and not surprisingly include knowledge of the subject matter, enthusiasm, and communication skills [2]. Is being a good educator a learned or innate skill? While many attributes of a good teacher may be innate the preponderance of data across many disciplines from athletics to medicine would suggest that being a good teacher is a skill that can be improved through thoughtful feedback, practice, and conscious reflection. Often this feedback may originate from an experienced mentor, colleague, or even the learner himself/herself. The fact that teaching is at least in part a learned skill argues that faculty development in education is important.

Surgical education has unique attributes that are different from traditional (nonsurgical) medical education. A good surgical educator is one who can most effectively convey and transmit medical knowledge and technical skill while demonstrating effective and compassionate patient care. This ability is likely developed longitudinally over time, and comes from a myriad of previous interactions as well as an inherent dedication and reverence to education. Effective surgical educators likely had effective surgical educators as mentors, and while the teaching techniques between individuals may be disparate, these interactions likely play a large role in modeling the commitment and dedication toward education.

It is difficult to determine how much an effective surgical educator learns "on the job"; however it is likely to be substantial. While many young faculty members enter the profession with an eagerness to teach and work with residents, the pressures of busy clinical practice can challenge this dedication. How residents are incorporated into clinical practice can also vary from faculty member to faculty member. All surgical educators have learned from their experience, have had to reevaluate their commitments from time to time, and have relied on feedback from trusted learners and mentors. A recent line of study has focused on observation or coaching in clinical teaching for surgeons [3]. This study highlighted the desire by surgical educators to be observed and receive feedback by faculty teaching experts, peers, and colleagues. The ability to enhance the learning curve to becoming an effective medical educator is no doubt an important area for future study.

ACGME Requirements

The ACGME sets the standards for GME programs in the United States. These standards have always included requirements for faculty qualifications and faculty involvement in the educational program. For instance the requirements state that the faculty must:

> *"devote sufficient time to the educational program to fulfill their supervisory and teaching responsibilities; and to demonstrate a strong interest in the education of residents."* and *"The faculty must establish and maintain an environment of inquiry and scholarship with an active research component [4, p. 5]."*

The ACGME also requires that faculty must be evaluated. Examples from the Common Program Requirements are:

> *"At least annually, the program must evaluate faculty performance as it relates to the educational program. These evaluations should include a review of the faculty's clinical teaching abilities, commitment to the educational program, clinical knowledge, professionalism, and scholarly activities. This evaluation must include at least annual written confidential evaluations by the residents"* [4, p. 21].

The ACGME has also recognized the importance of faculty development to the quality of resident education. Institutional requirements indicate that faculty development activities related to education are required:

> *"the program director and core faculty members engage in professional development applicable to their responsibilities as educational leaders* [5, p. 7].

The Orthopedic Residency Review Committee (RRC) has recently proposed a new requirement that will make regular faculty development activities and education necessary for all faculty. These activities should include the following areas: resident education, evaluation, feedback, mentoring, supervision, and teaching. The program must maintain documentation of faculty member participation in these activities, and provide it upon request. These requirements are fairly softly worded but they reflect that the RRC sees a need to further encourage faculty development. If this new requirement is approved, many programs will need to increase their effort to ensure that faculty members are periodically engaged in programs designed to enhance their teaching skills.

Venues of Teaching

Surgical faculty members must develop teaching skills in several important and varied environments. Some faculty are skilled educators in one area and have more difficulty in others. The following will briefly describe challenges that faculty must overcome to develop teaching skills in three different areas. As faculty seek to develop educational skills, separate attention to each of these areas is important, because they are different.

Teaching in Clinic

Developing patient care skills in the clinic is "home base" for most orthopedic practices, and teaching residents in this area is critically important. In most present-day academic centers there are significant challenges to optimal teaching in outpatient clinics. Residents usually prefer to be in the operating room, and rate clinic experiences heavily toward service. The clinician educators not only feel that there is inadequate time for teaching relative to the volume of clinical workload, but many feel that they have little control over the distribution and organization of this time [6]. Patients' perceptions of clinic encounters, including post-encounter surveys (e.g. Press Ganey), have further altered educational dynamics in outpatient settings. With increased emphasis and reporting of these metrics, the ability to be a teacher in an outpatient surgical clinic may be further jeopardized. Close examination of these trends will be warranted in the future to maintain an optimal learning environment. A balance will need to be obtained between the clinical service needs of the provider and patient and the educational needs of the student and/or resident learner.

A recent comprehensive review of educational research on ambulatory education highlighted two critical points. First, the environmental variables of a particular outpatient clinic such as (1) case mix in clinic, (2) pace of workload, (3) structured time for teaching, and (4) space for teaching have little if any impact on the overall ratings on the effectiveness of the teacher. Second, the behavior of teachers strongly influences the perceived success of the ambulatory educational experience. Effective teachers ask questions, show interest, define goals, demonstrate competence, and, most importantly, spend time with the learner [7]. In busy surgical clinics managing learner expectations by preparing the student/resident or fellow for what they may see or identify in a given patient encounter is extremely important, and then focusing on the specific teaching point, even if it is a small piece of information, has been most successful. Educational programs and mentor-driven guidance should highlight the importance and challenges inherent in educating residents in the clinic.

Teaching in the Operating Room

Residents spend the majority of their time in the operating room and need to learn numerous challenging skills to be technically competent at the end of training. The operating room is therefore a critically important area for faculty to develop educational skills. Numerous barriers to current surgical (intraoperative) education have been cited. These barriers including the decline in resident work hours, lack of structure or curricula in surgical training, intolerance of surgical error, and burdens of efficiency coupled with the financial realities of modern healthcare have all been felt to have had a negative impact on surgical training. Several important principles of orthopedic surgical training have been described [8]. These include the importance of teaching basic surgical skill or tasks outside of the operating room. Since the 2013 ACGME mandate, most programs now have surgical simulation programs. Young faculty should be encouraged or required to participate in these programs. This is a low-intensity area to develop and refine technical teaching skills. This area of surgical education will almost certainly grow during new faculty member's career and being involved from the beginning is very important.

In the actual operating room there are also significant educational challenges that will require faculty development and engagement. Teaching must occur in a heavily supervised environment that is efficient, and puts maximum emphasis on safe and high-quality patient care. Some basic teaching principles to convey to young faculty members include clarifying learning objectives and expectations prior to each operation, dividing the operation into component parts, deciding in advance which parts the resident will do and which parts will be done by the attending, and reviewing the results of each operation with the residents (debriefing) to identify lessons learned. Formal assessment of resident skill will increasingly be a part of faculty's responsibility in technical education, and faculty development will be necessary to get faculty to adapt and to embrace these impending new responsibilities.

Formal Teaching and Conference

The current focus on medical education is shifting away from traditional didactic lecture format and more toward clinically relevant case or simulation-based formats [9]. The ACGME mandates that residency programs provide regularly scheduled didactic sessions. The lecture format, while changing, remains a popular modality for inexpensive and accessible transfer of medical knowledge to large groups of medical students, residents, and fellows. However studies demonstrate only short-term gains in medical knowledge with poorer longer term retention from didactic venues [10]. Given the variability and retention of knowledge associated with traditional didactic lecture format, many have transitioned to largely case-based formats. How then do faculty best learn to teach in case-based formats? This can be challenging when young faculty are just entering into their chosen subspecialty field. Much of this development comes from seeing and watching the learning styles of respected and many times more senior educators. Watching an impassioned instructor discuss a particular patient, diagnosis, and treatment can provide invaluable lessons. Many times the most effective case-based educators demonstrate an uncanny ability to elicit level-in-training appropriate information from their audience, providing a challenging yet conducive environment for knowledge consolidation and transfer.

Development Resources for Faculty

A variety of resources exist for orthopedic surgical faculty educators. On a national level the ACGME provides a variety of courses, webinars, and online offerings on a number of educational related topics (ACGME.org). An example workshop currently being offered is *Developing Faculty Competencies in Assessment.* The American Academy of Orthopedic Surgery (AAOS) hosts an annual, long-standing, and intensive 3–4-day course, the Orthopedic Educators Course, which reviews a multitude of educational topics [11].

While it likely varies from institution to institution most academic medical centers also have Faculty Affairs Divisions or offices of Graduate Medical Education whose role is to facilitate faculty development in many of the previously discussed areas such as clinical teaching, scholarship and mentoring, and assessment. In addition to these offerings, most orthopedic departments have Chairs, Residency Directors, or Senior-respected expert educators who can provide advice, encouragement, and information on best educational practices.

For busy clinicians, particularly surgeons, taking valuable time away from other pursuits has a cost and needs to be meaningful. Emphasis on ongoing improvement in our collective abilities to teach and transmit knowledge to subsequent generations should be monitored and valued by our medical centers, departments, and profession. The ACGME and Orthopedic RRC have taken important steps forward in strongly encouraging core teaching faculty to participate in these development activities (see above). By sharing best practices and demonstrating a career-long commitment to education we will undoubtedly benefit our medical students, residents, and fellows.

Performance Assessment

Assessment of faculty is an important part of performance improvement. Residents must assess how their faculty members perform in providing education in the clinic, the OR, and other areas important to the residents. Feedback from these resident assessments is a critical part of the process of faculty development but how to achieve it has some challenges.

Resident assessment of faculty must be anonymous. This needs continual attention so the residents are assured that their evaluations are confidential and they are not subject to retaliation in anyway. We use both electronic and written forms since the residents seem to trust confidentiality in the latter more. In addition to electronic end-of-rotation evaluations, we use a separate yearly professionalism and education written form (Fig. 10.1). These evaluations provide both comparative numerical score and written assessments of faculty, both of which are important. We also use informal meetings with the residents by resident year to discuss various aspects of faculty-resident interaction. These allow the resident groups at the same level to discuss their experiences and openly discuss faculty performance. Faculty members are also assessed by the degree to which they adhere to department educational standards, such as weekly and team conference attendance; reviewing and meeting with residents prior to, during, and following the end of a rotation; completing resident evaluations; and participating in journal clubs, resident interviews, and various other aspects of the educational program. Feedback based on these assessments is a critical part of faculty development. The ACGME places responsibility on the Program Director for providing faculty feedback on their educational performance. A supportive and engaged chair is very helpful to maximize the benefit of feedback to faculty in their review. In our program, the department chairman reviews these resident evaluations and other aspects of

PROFESSIONALISM - EDUCATION 2015-2016

Evaluator: _______________________________

Evaluation of: _______________________________

Date: _______________________

Check the most appropriate box for each item regarding the professionalism of the individual at the top of the form. The three blank boxes represent unlabeled selections between almost never and nearly always

Professionalism

	Unable to Assess	Never	Almost never				Nearly always	Always
1. Listens well and responds appropriately	☐	☐	☐	☐	☐	☐	☐	☐
2. Inspires trust in patients, team members, and hospital staff	☐	☐	☐	☐	☐	☐	☐	☐
3. Demonstrates respect for all others, both in person and in indirect references	☐	☐	☐	☐	☐	☐	☐	☐
4. Acknowledges own limitations; accepts constructive feedback	☐	☐	☐	☐	☐	☐	☐	☐
5. Exemplifies professional behavior	☐	☐	☐	☐	☐	☐	☐	☐

6. Comments _______________________________

Education

	Unable to Assess	Never	Almost never				Nearly always	Always
7. Makes education a high priority in clinic	☐	☐	☐	☐	☐	☐	☐	☐
8. Makes education a high priority in the OR	☐	☐	☐	☐	☐	☐	☐	☐
9. Allows me to participate in surgery commensurate with my ability	☐	☐	☐	☐	☐	☐	☐	☐
10. Places education over service work in my daily activities	☐	☐	☐	☐	☐	☐	☐	☐
11. Participates in team and department conference in a way that improves education	☐	☐	☐	☐	☐	☐	☐	☐
12. Gives great lectures, case conferences or other formal teaching	☐	☐	☐	☐	☐	☐	☐	☐

13. Comments _______________________________

FIGURE 10.1 Faculty professionalism and education survey that has been utilized in the Department of Orthopedics and Rehabilitation at the University of Iowa. This 17-item survey is filled out by residents annually

Interaction With Residents and Students							
	Unable to Assess	Never	Almost never				Nearly always	Always
14. Treats residents and students with respect and dignity								
15. Works to see that I adhere to work hour guidelines and other departmental rules	☐	☐	☐	☐	☐	☐	☐	☐
16. Minimizes my requirements for service activities (late dictating, call backs etc)	☐	☐	☐	☐	☐	☐	☐	☐
17. Comments								

FIGURE 10.1 (continued)

faculty performance in the educational program individually with faculty members. Specific educational goals are set on a yearly basis.

Faculty Motivation

There are many, and oftentimes conflicting, demands placed upon academic orthopedic surgeons. On the one hand being a good educator can be extremely rewarding, but at other times it can lead to or feel like an inefficient use of valuable time. How then do we motivate educational initiatives and performance? Rewards, recognition, and even small financial incentives for performance can help to motivate faculty and emphasize the importance of the educational mission. Departments should be open and transparent about the educational expectations and opportunities within their unique environments. Our department has developed, maintained, and modified an educational scorecard for faculty that highlights the importance of many things that are considered to be valuable within our educational environment. It is based on a point system for various educational activities (Fig. 10.2). It may also be used to determine which faculty may be best suited to work with residents, and those who would be better suited to work independently. This is often a motivating

a

Educational Activities Scorecard	Points
Conferences	
Monday	1
Tuesday	2
Wednesday	2
Senior Residents Day - Friday	4
Senior Residents Day - Saturday	2
Shrine	1
Other	1
Milestone Evaluations	
Timely filled out on all residents (within 2 weeks)	1
Met and provided feedback with residents (within 2 weeks)	2
Filled out late and did not meet with resident	-3
Resident Recruitment	
Resident application screening committee	3
Participated in resident interviews	3
AGME Required Committees	
PEC Committee	2
CCC Committee	2
Medical School Education	
M3, M4 roation lectures	1
FCP4 Lectures	2
Small group teaching (entire academic year)	1
ECE Mentoring (entire academic year)	2
Medical student interviews	1
Other	
Suguical skills teaching in the PGY1 course	3
Attendance at journal club	1
Dir Res/Senior Resident Day Dir	10
Medical student direcor	10
Senior Resident Day/Research Comember	1
IOJ editor	5
Resident Evaluation of Teaching	

FIGURE 10.2 (**a**) Spreadsheet noting activities recorded in an educational scorecard. (**b**) Chart representing the spectrum of faculty performances utilizing an educational scorecard at our institution

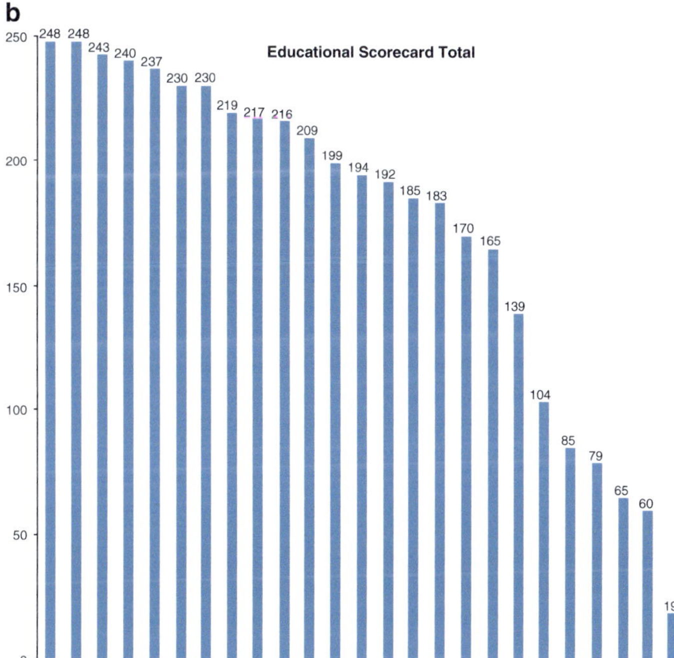

FIGURE 10.2 (continued)

incentive but can potentially lead to a restriction of resident-faculty interactions if warranted.

The Role of Mentorship

The importance of mentorship of young faculty cannot be overstated. Mentoring may be defined as a relationship, formal or informal, between a novice and one or more senior persons in the field for the purposes of career and personal development and preparation for leadership [12]. While relatively few studies have specifically looked at mentorship in orthopedics several themes do recur. For younger faculty members it is important that there is an understanding of the departmental practices and norms. In other words, what are the expectations of good educational "citizenship" within a department? For many it may seem like the answer to this question would be obvious; however be the complexities of a busy academic orthopedic department the opportunities and expectations can be extremely variable. For example: How does one balance a busy adult reconstruction practice with demands for didactic instruction for the college of medicine? This is just one example of a myriad of trade-offs that a junior faculty member may encounter. Advice on how to incorporate residents into surgical cases, how to balance education with practice efficiency, and how to teach in clinic are examples of activities where open discussion with a senior mentor can be very valuable. Perhaps one of the most important aspects of the mentor–mentee relationship is the usefulness of feedback. While feedback can take many forms, from formalized annual or semiannual reporting to critical appraisal of research or academic pursuits, the genuine commitment of the mentor to the development of the mentee is paramount to success.

Stages of a Career

Faculty members at a teaching institution typically emphasize and focus on different things during different stages of their career. As a career progresses, a faculty member's practice focus may narrow and their referral base increase. Time spent on research may be more or less at different times during a career. Faculty members may evolve into leadership roles either locally at the medical center or in national organizations. However, a focus on education must span all these stages of a career. Early in their career faculty identify their roles in the department. They need to develop teaching materials to deliver conferences and case-based sessions. This is a good time for them to become engaged in the overall educational program of the department by becoming a member of education committees. Program Evaluation Committee and Clinical Competency Committee often need willing and hardworking new faculty members. Most programs will have one or both of a resident selection committee or resident research committee. Medical school curriculum and selection committees are time consuming but may be rewarding. It is during this time that mentorship is most important. The chairman, program director, or other senior faculty member should fill this role.

Mid-career faculty members have different challenges. Their practice may have become quite busy, and they may be involved in various national activities. These things may impinge on education, and worse may lead the faculty member to push the residents toward service to support their busy practices. The educational skills learned early in their career may have been pushed into the background. These faculty need to be reminded of the purpose and mission of the department. Accurate assessment of faculty performance and feedback is important.

Senior faculty members are often mature educators that bring a wealth of experience and wisdom to teaching sessions. Hopefully, their skills can be utilized to assist in mentoring junior faculty or residents. The challenges for these faculty members often lie in adapting to new educational initiatives, such as new milestone evaluations, electronic evaluations of resident rotation performance, or surgical skill. For instance providing timely resident assessment forms or joining CCC or PEC may be issues for senior faculty.

All of these characterizations about career stages should be considered generalities that do not apply to all faculty members. Some faculty members are passionate about the educational process throughout their careers despite other changes, and others find it difficult to engage residents in their practice from the beginning.

Summary and Conclusions

Faculty development has become an increasingly important part of educational programs. Residency training is gradually changing from the traditional apprenticeship model, and the educational expectations of faculty members are changing. As pressures on faculty have increased the need for formal and informal development to help faculty achieve educational goals has become very important. Assessment and feedback to faculty and mentorship are important parts of good development programs. Faculty engagement with education evolves during a career, and the needs for development change. Faculty development and education are likely to be required by the Orthopedic RRC, but good programs already have faculty education and development programs in place to assure that the program faculty provide the appropriate educational environment.

References

1. Simon MA. The clinician educator. J Bone Joint Surg Am. 2005;87(9):2131–2.
2. Singh S, Pai DR, Sinha NK, Kaur A, Soe HH, Barua A. Qualities of an effective teacher: what do medical teachers think? BMC Med Educ. 2013;13:128.
3. Peyre SE, Frankl SE, Thorndike M, Breen EM. Observation of clinical teaching: interest in a faculty development program for surgeons. J Surg Educ. 2011;68(5):372–6.
4. Requirements AOP. http://www.acgme.org/Portals/0/PFAssets/ProgramRequirements/260_orthopaedic_surgery_2016.pdf.
5. Requirements AI. https://www.acgme.org/Portals/0/PDFs/FAQ/InstitutionalRequirements_07012015.pdf. Page 7.
6. McGee SR, Irby DM. Teaching in the outpatient clinic. Practical tips. J Gen Intern Med. 1997;12 Suppl 2:S34–40.
7. Irby DM. Teaching and learning in ambulatory care settings: a thematic review of the literature. Acad Med. 1995;70(10):898–931.
8. Pinney SJ, Mehta S, Pratt DD, Sarwark JF, Campion E, Blakemore L, et al. Orthopaedic surgeons as educators. Applying the principles of adult education to teaching orthopaedic residents. J Bone Joint Surg Am. 2007;89(6):1385–92.
9. Wolf BR, Britton CL. How orthopaedic residents perceive educational resources. Iowa Orthop J. 2013;33:185–90.
10. Sawatsky AP, Zickmund SL, Berlacher K, Lesky D, Granieri R. Understanding resident learning preferences within an internal medicine noon conference lecture series: a qualitative study. J Grad Med Educ. 2014;6(1):32–8.
11. Course AE. http://www.aaos.org/calendar/event/?productId=9235810.
12. Wilson FC. Mentoring in orthopaedics: an evolving need for nurture. J Bone Joint Surg Am. 2004;86-A(5):1089–91.

Chapter 11
Elements of a Successful Program

M. Daniel Wongworawat, Martin J. Morrison III,
and Hasan M. Syed

Having the Right Team: Getting a Good Match

A successful residency program starts out with building the right team of teachers and learners. While composition of the faculty may fluctuate, the piece that changes year to year is the class of incoming residents. Applicants seem to increase in competitiveness, where the number of publications, presentations, and abstracts more than doubled since 2007. Similarly, the United States Medical Licensing Examination (USMLE) Step-1 and Step-2 scores have seen an increase, now averaging 245 and 251, respectively. However, the students who apply and match to orthopaedic surgery programs still represent the same sector of each graduating class and the percentage who hold Alpha Omega Alpha (AOA) election has remained fairly constant [1].

Selecting from this highly qualified pool of applicants is a complicated task. With a large number of variables to evaluate, the selection criteria that are strongly correlated with

M.D. Wongworawat, MD (✉)
M.J. Morrison III, MD • H.M. Syed, MD
Loma Linda University Medical Center,
11406 Loma Linda Drive, Suite 218, Loma Linda, CA 92354, USA
e-mail: dwongworawat@llu.edu; mmorrison@llu.edu; hsyed@llu.edu

© Springer International Publishing AG 2018

P.J. Dougherty, B.L. Joyce (eds.), *The Orthopedic Educator*,
DOI 10.1007/978-3-319-62944-5_11

resident performance are USMLE Step-2 score, the number of honors in medical school clerkships, and AOA election [2–4]. USMLE Step-1 scores have also been shown to have a strong correlation with passing ABOS Step 1 Examination [5]. USMLE Step-1 and Step-2 scores show the applicant's ability to apply medical knowledge. The number of honors makes intuitive sense, since doing well in other specialties reflects one's ability to go above and beyond even if not interested in that field; these findings echo an earlier report, where performance in clinical clerkships most predicts resident performance [6]. Finally, election to AOA embodies academics, service, leadership, and scholarly activity. Several years after their initial recommendations, there was repeated emphasis on the initial recommendations of the American Orthopaedic Association Steering Committee on resident selection criteria which focused on five domains: (1) mechanics of resident selection, (2) assessment of cognitive ability, (3) assessment of motor ability, (4) affective domain or non-cognitive factors, and (5) assessment of "dropouts" [7]. Clearly, the first two items have been studied vigorously, but remaining domains are still works in progress.

Our program found that a practical application involves first screening applicants based on quantifiable factors: USMLE scores, number of honors, number of research activities, and AOA election. After the initial screening, we invite applicants for interview. Because structured interviews with anchored scales are more reliable [8], we have found utility in having multiple evaluators grading each domain (such as teamwork), each evaluator judging more than one domain (such as leadership skill and ethical reasoning), and using scales with preprinted definitions. We derive our preliminary rank list using both objective preinterview factors and subjective interview ratings. Starting with this first ranking, the selection committee makes minor adjustments to create the final rank list.

Faculty members represent another crucial part of the team, but there is little literature guidance on how to select the program's core faculty. The Accreditation Council for

Graduate Medical Education (ACGME) provides guidelines that the faculty must devote sufficient time and demonstrate a strong interest in education, maintain a good learning environment, and meet licensure and certification requirements; for every four residents, there must be at least one full-time faculty member. Additionally, faculty members should be committed to promoting an environment of inquiry and scholarship [9]. Each person will contribute something different to the educational program. For instance, various faculty members will be involved in conducting original research, writing chapters, presenting at meetings, or participating in national organizations. All these activities complement the program. Additionally, having at least one faculty member for each subspecialty area is helpful.

Case Volume

Variability in case volume, during residency training, may contribute to differences in experience and, potentially, to qualifications upon graduation or entrance to fellowship training. While case logs were required by the ACGME, there were few guidelines about minimum surgeries in specific categories, and large variability in procedures per category existed among graduating residents. One study found that there was a significant gap in adult case volume between residents in the 10th and the 90th percentiles [10]. Similarly, another study of upper extremity cases found wide variance in case volume between the top and bottom 10% of residents, where the difference was more than fivefold. The authors suggested that these variances likely have educational implications [11]. Case volume disparity has been reported for arthroscopy experience as well, but overall, volume for arthroscopic cases has increased over the study periods [12].

To somewhat control for disparity in case volume, the ACGME updated the case log requirements in 2014, where resident case numbers must be at least 1000 total cases but no more than 3000 total cases. Even so, this mandate reflects a potential threefold difference in experience. Additionally, to ensure minimum exposure to certain surgeries, the ACGME established minimums as stratified by case type (Table 11.1): knee arthroscopy (30 cases), shoulder arthroscopy (20), anterior cruciate ligament reconstruction (10), total hip arthroplasty (30), total knee arthroplasty (30), hip fracture surgery (30), carpal tunnel release (10), spine decompression and fusion (15), ankle fracture fixation (15), closed reduction of the forearm and wrist (20), ankle and foot arthrodesis (5), supracondylar humerus percutaneous fixation (5), femoral and tibial shaft fracture fixation (25), all pediatric procedures (200), and all oncology procedures (10) [13].

The effects of case log minimums have yet to be seen. In a recent survey, residents consider case minimums as an effective monitoring tool of resident progress, but surgical ability

TABLE 11.1 Minimum case numbers by category

Knee arthroscopy	30
Shoulder arthroscopy	20
Anterior cruciate ligament reconstruction	10
Total hip arthroplasty	30
Total knee arthroplasty	30
Hip fractures	30
Carpal tunnel release	10
Spine decompression/posterior spine fusion	15
Ankle fracture fixation	15
Closed reduction forearm/wrist	20
Ankle and hind and mid-foot arthrodeses	5
Supracondylar humerus percutaneous treatment	5
Operative treatment of femoral and tibial shaft fractures	25
All pediatric procedures	200
All oncology	10

is difficult to evaluate based on minimums alone [14]. There is much variability in clinical exposure to surgeries, and case volume is not the only determinant of training quality, since case complexity, breadth of pathology, and teaching quality influence the learner's experience [15]. While using minimums as a benchmark for surgical ability is crude at best, the objective structured assessment of technical skills (OSATS) and associated checklist scores aim to bring validity [16]. However, the improved validity of OSATS scoring does not necessarily translate into better surgical results [17, 18].

Institutional Support

Among the program requirements for orthopaedic surgery residency, the sponsoring institution must assume responsibility for the program, and this responsibility includes oversight of all participating training sites [9]. The sponsoring institution must also have accredited programs in general surgery, internal medicine, and pediatrics, so that the residents are able to have an interdisciplinary experience.

In addition to the oversight of training sites, the institution is responsible for ensuring adequate time and availability of the Program Director (PD) and support staff. The PD must have sufficient protected time and institutional financial support so that administrative and educational responsibilities can be met. In addition, the Program Coordinator is responsible for assisting in providing effective administration. For large programs, where there are more than 20 residents, additional administrative personnel should be provided.

Institutional support extends to educational resources. These resources include specialty-specific full-text journals and reference books accessible by electronic means. The most common access is through Internet log-in, where residents at remote affiliated sites have the ability to readily view articles and texts. Additionally, institutional support includes making sure that there are adequate workspaces for the residents, with access to computer resources for research, writing manuscripts, preparing presentations, and upkeep of portfolios. Most programs incorporate anatomy sessions with cadaver dissections, focusing on surgical approaches. While few programs include formal microsurgical training, we give our residents 40 h of instruction on mice. More recently, with the additional requirement of basic surgical skill instruction, dedicated space must be available, and future requirements may include simulation training.

Beyond institutional support, orthopaedic departments also provide additional benefits to residents. More than three-quarters of residents receive discretionary funds and funding to attend conferences. A recent survey found that most of these funds came from the department, followed by funding from the hospital or institution. Nearly all programs provided meal stipends, and the majority gave free parking, gym benefits, surgical loupes, and maternity/paternity leave beyond vacation time [19].

Research Support

Resident research is an essential component of an orthopaedic residency program [20]. Towards this end, several elements of support are necessary to help achieve meaningful research productivity. A mechanism for resident research funding at a basic level, institutional review board application submission, and collaboration with other laboratories/departments provide for an environment where resident research can be successful [21].

Within our institution, initial funding for approved orthopaedic projects comes from a departmental fund that creates a small budget for residents to start pilot studies and/or purchase material for their research. In addition, residents are encouraged to apply for research grants available nationally. Within our department, there is an administrator who assists with obtaining approval from the Institutional Review Board (IRB) and works with Grants Management. The institution also provides formal statistical consultation to assist with resident research.

Multidisciplinary collaboration across departments allows for better resource utilization for conducting research. We have a biomechanics laboratory with a dedicated researcher to help residents set up appropriate mechanical testing models. In addition, the Research Director maintains contacts with various departments such as radiology, physiatry, and neurosurgery, as well as basic science labs at the institutional level allowing residents to utilize bench space and obtain basic science expertise for their projects.

Several members within the department are essential to assisting residents with their research. At our institution, the members that form the Orthopedic Research Committee (ORC) consist of a research-oriented orthopaedic clinician who acts as the Research Director, the Program Director, all residents on research rotations, a basic scientist specialized in biomechanics, and administrative personnel who assist with the research database and IRB applications. The ORC meets monthly to review all research proposal presentations, discuss logistical issues pertaining to research, and plan for the annual department research seminar.

Being a Successful Program Director

Responsibilities of the Program Director

The first priority of the Program Director (PD) is to ensure the quality of education for all residents at all participating sites. Quality of education includes both didactic and clinical components. At each participating site where residents rotate, the PD approves the local director as well as approves the selection of all new faculty members associated with the program. Continued participation of program faculty members is based on routine faculty evaluations completed by residents after each rotation.

To safeguard the learning environment, the PD must make sure that ACGME and institutional policies and procedures are implemented. This includes ensuring adequate supervision at each participating site, monitoring policy, adherence to duty hours, adjusting schedules to mitigate fatigue, and providing access to online educational resources [9].

The PD is also responsible for monitoring data for process improvement. This information comes by way of evaluations and surveys: evaluations of residents; the residents' evaluations of faculty members, rotations, and program; and past graduates' evaluations of the program. These will be detailed later in the chapter.

With the many varied responsibilities of the Program Director, a calendar is helpful. Our program developed this calendar to aid in staying on track (Table 11.2). The keystone meeting is the Residency Program Evaluation Committee (RPEC), which is convened on a semiannual basis; all evaluation data are reviewed and recommendations for program improvement are made. We also have other committees that enhance program administration. Twice a year, we hold a Resident Forum, where the PD and Associate Program Director (APD) meet with all the residents to discuss any suggestions and concerns. Then, between these meetings, the PD meets with the Resident Representation Committee (RRC)—comprised of one member elected from each class—on an as-needed basis to solicit comments and to handle problems. As required by the ACGME, we also convene the Clinical Competency Committee (CCC) ahead of each semiannual Residency Program Evaluation Committee. The CCC reviews data from each resident's evaluations and pegs performance to the Milestones [22]. While we have not implemented this practice, resident self-assessment using the Milestones may provide personal insight, and one study found that residents were able to successfully self-assess, with improving proficiency over time [23].

Building a Team

A successful residency program requires a well-functioning team, and the key components of this team are the Associate Program Director (APD), Program Coordinator, and core faculty members.

TABLE 11.2 Calendar of program director tasks

July	• Publish important dates for the academic year
	• Publish improvement implementation plan, based on action items derived from the June semiannual Residency Program Evaluation Committee
	• Run basic surgical skill course for incoming residents
	• ABOS modules for incoming residents
	• Arrange fracture course for junior residents
	• Oversee fellowship application process for new PGY-4 residents
August	• Conduct 360° evaluations, including patient surveys, case management surveys, nursing evaluations
September	• Assemble Resident Selection Committee
	• Convene Resident Representation Committee
November	• Orient members of the Resident Selection Committee
	• Draft agenda for the semiannual Residency Program Evaluation Committee
	• Draft agenda for the Resident Forum
	• Convene Resident Representation Committee
	• Conduct 360° evaluations
	• Convene Clinical Competency Committee
	• Remind senior residents about graduation requirements
December	• Consider nomination of one or more residents to the Alpha Omega Alpha Honor Medical Society
	• Conduct the semiannual Residency Program Evaluation Committee
	• Meet with individual residents for semiannual review

(continued)

TABLE 11.2 (continued)

January	• Interview residency applicants and submit rank order list
	• Arrange board review course for senior residents
February	• Convene Resident Representation Committee
	• Conduct 360° evaluations
	• Finalize details for the Orthopaedic Research Seminar
March	• Send out goals and objectives to all services for updates and revisions
	• Solicit from faculty members any potential changes or suggestions to current policies and procedures
	• Select Program Resident Representative for American Orthopaedic Association Resident Leadership Forum
April	• Draft conference schedule for next academic year
	• Plan residency graduation events
May	• Update Residency Program Policies and Procedures and send out to faculty members for review
	• Draft agenda for the Residency Program Evaluation Committee
	• Draft agenda for resident forum
	• Invite guest professor for next year's Orthopaedic Research Seminar
	• Solicit evaluations from faculty members, residents, and past graduates regarding the training program
	• Convene Resident Representation Committee
	• Conduct 360° evaluations
	• Convene clinical competency committee

TABLE 11.2 (continued)

June	• Perform exit interviews with senior residents
	• Conduct the semiannual Residency Program Evaluation Committee
	• Meet with individual residents for semiannual review
	• Meet with Chair to discuss faculty development and advancement
	• Re-administration of ABOS modules for completing PGY-1s

Associate Program Director

The Associate Program Director (APD), along with the Program Director (PD), carries authority and accountability in maintaining the residency program [24], particularly in programs with greater than 20 residents. The APD serves to assist, and, at times, stand in the stead of, the PD. The APD allows for continuous access for the residents to the staff and core faculty of the Residency Program. In addition to being the liaison between the residents and the program, the APD also serves to further aid in core faculty development within the residency. The APD collaborates with the PD to optimize scheduling and ensure adherence to ACGME policies, recommendations, and deadlines.

Program Coordinator

The role of the Program Coordinator is becoming increasingly important. From initially being more clerical, the increased requirements of the ACGME—from the Outcome Project to Milestones implementation—have driven the Coordinator's role to be more managerial. One survey found a high level of day-to-day managerial oversight of all aspects of residency training, and often, there are additional responsibilities for faculty development and other business [25]. Because of the complexities of managing a residency, of assisting the Program Director in assuring compliance with current policies and maintaining accreditation, we recommend professional certification of the Program Coordinator. Training Administrators of Graduate Medical Education (TAGME) certification assures knowledge in key knowledge content areas, including milestones and competencies, evaluations, procedure logs, and other ACGME-related regulations. Engagement in the Association of Residency Coordinators in Orthopaedic Surgery (ARCOS) provides a forum for support and enables the coordinator to keep up to date with current recommendations and best practices.

Faculty Members

The biggest recent change, and perhaps a challenge, in educating the program's core faculty members came with the advent of competency-based education. To many faculty members who trained in the pre-competency era, much of the terminology remains nebulous. For instance, despite advances in defining systems-based practice competency, a recent study of orthopaedic educators and residents found that the teaching of this domain is highly inconsistent, and formal assessment rarely happens [26]. However, current guidelines mandate that training be mapped to core competencies, and with work-hour limits available for clinical training, rotations based on competency, rather than on time, may be the answer in maximizing the use of available hours [27].

While all faculty members have spent their lifetime in education, few are trained in education. One successful and highly recommended faculty development program is sponsored by the American Academy of Orthopaedic Surgeons (AAOS). We encourage each of our faculty members to attend this week-long AAOS Course for Orthopaedic Educators at least once. Upon returning, each faculty is given an opportunity to share points learned during a departmental meeting. These experiences enrich the faculty member, giving each one a better understanding of competency-based training, a sense of community with other orthopaedic educators, and tools for setting expectations, providing feedback to residents, and working with problem residents. Additionally, we invite speakers for Grand Rounds, and educational topics (such as recognizing resident fatigue) are covered several times a year. At the institutional level, our GME office holds a 1-day retreat for the Program Director, the Associate Program Director, and the Program Coordinator, where didactic sessions are mixed with case-based discussions on topics pertaining to resident education.

Meeting the ACGME Standards

Graduate Performance

Ultimately, residency training produces graduates who are able to independently practice orthopaedic surgery without supervision. While this is difficult to fully assess, there are several measures of graduate performance. The American Board of Orthopaedic Surgery (ABOS) provides Part I and Part II scores to the programs, and the Part I scores are subdivided into domains. How a resident performs on the Orthopaedic In-Training Examination relates to ABOS Part I scores [5, 28–30], but certification is contingent on passing the both Parts I and II. One benchmark is to compare program pass rates to the national average, which is between 79 and 88% [31].

Another measure of program effectiveness is obtained by simply asking past graduates questions about their training and where gaps in training may be. Ahead of our academic year-end Residency Program Evaluation Committee meeting, we survey our recent graduates. Questions relate to the training received, such as preparation for handling clinical situations and surgical cases, breadth of orthopaedic knowledge, and skills for systems-based practice. Finally, past graduates are asked about skills acquired that promote the habit of lifelong learning and improvement. Our program reviews past-graduate responses on an annual basis. We utilize this data to improve areas of perceived weakness and reinforce areas which are strong.

Resident Survey

Around the third quarter of the academic year (starting January), the ACGME requires that at least 70% of residents in a particular program complete surveys about their educational and clinical experiences. The confidential responses are aggregated to the program level, and the Program Director is provided these responses [32]. Content areas include compliance with duty hours, supervision and instruction from faculty, opportunities for and satisfaction with evaluations, satisfaction with educational content, availability of educational resources and accessibility of medical records, and effectiveness in promoting a culture of patient safety through interprofessional teams [33].

In addition to the formal ACGME survey, we solicit evaluations from each resident. At the end of each rotation, the residents evaluate the faculty members and the rotation. Rotation evaluations are based on how well each core competency is taught and modeled. The six core competencies are Patient Care, Medical Knowledge, Practice-based Learning, Professionalism, Interpersonal and Communication Skills, and Systems-based Practice. Additionally, we solicit open comments for areas needing improvement. These evaluations are collected during the course of the year, and rather than presenting the results to the faculty members after each rotation, aggregated responses are provided at year-end. This serves to protect anonymity and ensure confidentiality. Because of this, it allows for more sincere responses from residents.

Faculty Survey

Similar to the Resident Survey, the ACGME surveys faculty members once a year during the third academic quarter.

At least 60% of faculty members must complete the survey [34]. Content domains include supervision and teaching (sufficient time to supervise residents, and faculty performance is evaluated), educational content (milestones achievement, clinical content in various settings, training for fatigue management), resources (faculty development, process to handle grievances), patient safety (handoffs, quality improvement), and teamwork (communication skills); the survey items are based on the current academic year [35]. Aggregated reports become available to the Program Director and the Designated Institutional Official after the survey closes if the minimum response rate of 60% is reached.

In addition to the ACGME survey, we conduct an internal survey towards the end of each academic year. In preparation for the June Residency Program Evaluation Committee meeting, faculty members are sent a questionnaire designed to elicit program effectiveness as stratified by the core competencies of Patient Care, Medical Knowledge, Practice-based Learning, Professionalism, Interpersonal and Communication Skills, and Systems-based Practice. Questions pertaining to these competencies relate to rotation design and exposure to outpatient clinics, inpatient services, and operative care; Grand Rounds and core didactic conferences; case-based and specialty-specific conferences; patient safety and morbidity-mortality conferences; patient communication and cultural competency; and coordination of care and quality improvement initiatives.

One of the more effective ways is to incorporate a narrative section in the faculty survey. We have found that thoughtful suggestions for program improvement come from these open-ended questions, as these responses do not fit neatly into checkboxes or on Likert scales.

Procedure Logs

The ACGME-updated case log guidelines require residents to complete between 1000 and 3000 cases by the end of training. As part of training, each resident logs surgical experiences. While some surgeries may entail multiple Current Procedural

Terminology (CPT) codes, one code is designated as the primary procedure, but additional codes (such as in multilevel spine surgery) are entered as well to reflect the complexity of the case. Additionally, for each case, the resident is designated as Level 1 or Level 2, where the former level is for primary involvement in performing key portions of the case or in teaching more junior residents, and the latter level is for assisting or in participating in non-key portions of the surgery. If the CPT code maps to a specific defined case category (Table 11.1), credit is applied towards that category's minimum. Additional areas of interest are pediatric patients (younger than 17 years), oncology, and microsurgery [36].

Ensuring timely logging of cases can be a challenge. Ideally, residents should log cases immediately following surgery or by the end of the day. Our program allows a 2-week period, after which the resident will be pulled from service until case logs are brought up to date. We review logs on a quarterly basis, and if large disparities are seen, rotation or daily assignments are rearranged. At each semiannual face-to-face evaluation with the residents, each individual is given a review of case log progress; deidentified data from other residents are also shown, so that the resident can self-evaluate against the comparable class cohort. Starting with the year-end evaluation at the end of postgraduate year (PGY) 4, the resident's case log progress is compared with the published minimums for each category (Table 11.1); if deficiencies are anticipated, corrective action can be taken by making rotation adjustments.

Metrics for Program Evaluation

We aggregate data for review. Sources include performance on standardized tests, ACGME communications, and surveys.

Drilling down on data from standardized tests, we review the breakdown of how residents and past graduates perform in each domain. The Orthopaedic In-Training Examination

(OITE) report includes aggregate data for the entire program as well as by training year with comparisons to the national norm. This information can be useful for programmatic changes. For instance, if the junior-level residents consistently score lower in the domain of basic science while the senior-level residents score higher, changes can be made to introduce more basic science teaching into the earlier years. We also review aggregated and deidentified Boards Part I scores as stratified by domains, and we modify our didactic program in response.

Communication from the ACGME regarding accreditation status may contain areas of concern or suggestions for improvement. ACGME survey results also contain valuable information about duty-hour violations and teaching effectiveness. Working with faculty members and resident representation, improvement plans are devised.

We also review internal data. In addition to evaluations from faculty, residents, and past graduates, we track resident and faculty presentations and publications. Publications associated with PubMed identifiers (PMID) are of particular interest, as these are specifically tracked and reported in our Annual Performance Evaluation and also reported to the ACGME's Accreditation Data System (ADS).

Annual Program Evaluation

At the end of each academic year, after the June meeting of the Residency Program Evaluation Committee, we prepare the Annual Program Evaluation for our Graduate Medical Education Committee (GMEC). Our Annual Program Evaluation is divided into several sections.

First, we provide a review of previous assessments. We report how we addressed concerns provided by the ACGME's Orthopaedic Residency Review Committee. If our GMEC had provided any oversight concerns or focused self-study requirements, responses are documented here. The top three improvement action plans from the year-end Residency

Program Evaluation Committee are reported. We also review faculty development efforts in the previous academic year and the residency program's curriculum.

The next section of the Annual Program Evaluation reviews data. This includes procedure logs and survey responses from recent graduates. Then, we evaluate our recent residents' pass rate for the ABOS Part I and Part II Examinations, and if the pass rate is below the national average, we devise and implement an improvement plan. We also review scholarly activity, both for residents and faculty members; in particular, we track the number of published articles that have a PubMed identifier (PMID). Next, we review resident involvement in projects relating to quality improvement, process improvement, patient safety, and healthcare disparities. Our residency also reports the Clinical Competency Committee (CCC) process and confirms that residents receive summative face-to-face evaluations at least twice a year. Finally, we explain the ACGME Faculty and Resident Surveys' results and consider improvements that might be implemented.

Planning ahead, the Annual Program Evaluation includes three improvement areas for the upcoming academic year. And as part of ensuring program viability, our GMEC requires succession planning; usually, the next in line is the Associate Program Director.

Tips for Success

Be Positive

Making the work environment an enjoyable place allows residents to work in a stress-free environment. The task of learning all that is expected during residency is a daunting process. While a hierarchy clearly exists, residents will become colleagues for far longer than they are trainees. Understanding this relationship and acknowledging residents as future colleagues promote a mutually rewarding relationship. Residents often choose mentors based on the behavior that they intend to model. In order to appeal to a broad and heterogeneous group of residents, it is vital to have faculty that model positive behavior among each other, with patients, and as teachers to serve as mentors for all types of adult learners.

Meet with Residents on a Regular Basis

We conduct three types of regular meetings with the residents: individual resident semiannual evaluation meetings, Resident Forum meetings, and senior resident exit interviews.

Individual resident meetings are held twice a year. After the Residency Program Evaluation Committee meetings of December and June for each academic year, individual face-to-face appointments are held between the Program Director and each resident. We review case log metrics and milestones achievements. These semiannual summative evaluations incorporate end-of-rotation evaluations, test scores, and 360° feedback from staff. Additional metrics may be available from objective structured clinical examinations (OSCEs) and OSATs [37–39]. There may be times for added meetings with the resident. One example is in the context of remediation. Sometimes, there are reasons for remediation, such as lack of professionalism or scoring below a threshold on the Orthopaedic In-Training Examination (OITE). Professionalism issues may present as problems on 360°evaluations or from direct reports by staff; while commitment to the virtues of virtues such as fidelity, trust, benevolence, intellectual honesty, courage, compassion, and truthfulness can be taught in lectures, modeling outside of the classroom is probably more important [40, 41]. Professionalism lapses should be handled on a case-by-case basis. For medical knowledge assessment, our program sets a threshold at 40th percentile for the OITE, below which the resident is placed in a remediation reading program. A report on General Surgery programs found that residency programs where the Program Director was actively involved in remediation mentorship and tracked resident reading performed better on in-training examinations [42].

We also hold Resident Forum meetings twice a year. These meetings are attended by all residents, the Program Director, and the Associate Program Director, with the purpose of giving the residents an open voice to express concerns. While the junior residents may have more specific suggestions, we found that senior resident presence is helpful in guiding the discussion, sometimes quelling issues brought up by junior residents. Action plans are drafted as a result of these discussions.

Senior resident exit interviews are especially important for program development. The voice of these graduating residents embodies all the years of residency training. Because these residents have gone through the entire educational process, they are able to provide a perspective from the end of the training journey [43]. Their voice is also one of authenticity, because they are no longer encumbered by the complexities of politics, by fear of repercussion, or by considerations of personal gain. Therefore, we take comments from the exit interviews seriously.

Meet with Faculty on a Regular Basis

While there are many faculty group meetings throughout the year to assess the residency and the faculty on the whole, the Chairman also conducts semiannual one-on-one meetings with individual faculty members to address progress, comments, and concerns. In addition to providing regular 360 degree feedback, the goal of these meetings is improvement in areas of concern as voiced by the faculty, residents, or ACGME-derived metrics. Additional meetings are held between faculty and the Chairman, Program Director, or Associate Program Director on an as-needed basis. Emphasis is always placed on resident requirements mandated by the ACGME.

Developing Resident Research

The goal of resident research is to instill in trainees the capacity to critically evaluate medical literature, surgical research, and other scholarly activities [20]. Critical to teaching these skills is having a research program structure, time, curriculum, and requirements. Providing a team-based structure has been shown to increase research productivity and give a better learning environment for residents [21].

At our institution, residents are provided dedicated research time during PGY-3 and PGY-4 training. Prior to engaging in any research activity, residents must obtain approval by formally presenting the research idea to the ORC. These ideas are generated by the residents themselves or selected from the departmental research idea database. Approval for the project is based on scientific methodology and clinical relevance. Residents are required to have at least one hypothesis testing project, but are encouraged to have two such projects. If only one hypothesis testing project is completed, two additional projects are required such as case reports, review articles, or book chapters. Residents are required to submit the research manuscripts to peer-reviewed journal in order to receive credit. If the first submission is not accepted, a second submission attempt is required to a different journal.

We have found it to be critical to have a Web-based database that keeps an inventory of all resident research projects and a separate research idea database, where ideas generated by faculty members and residents are logged and made available after an initial vetting process by the Research Director. The Research Director maintains this database and periodically contacts the residents to monitor progress.

The culmination of resident research is the presentation of such projects at the annual orthopaedic research seminar. A visiting professor is invited to be the moderator for this event. In addition residents are encouraged and funded to present their research at regional and national meetings.

Summary

Many elements compose a successful residency program team. This learner-focused team places the residents at the center, and one of the most important pieces begins with resident selection. We can describe the ideal resident (bright, skilled, hardworking, good teammate), but the ideal selection process remains elusive. Once matriculated, the residents need an orchestrated learning environment, where institutional support is rich and departmental resources complete. Within the department, creating an environment for scholarly activity involves building a team and setting up a system to encourage resident research with appropriate oversight. Personnel resources within the department include the Program Director, Associate Program Director, Research Director, Program Coordinator, and all core faculty members; each role requires adequate training and knowledge of role expectations. Finally, connecting all the pieces—residents, faculty members, staff, department, and institution—requires effective assessments and confidential evaluations. It is through tabulating objective metrics and considering subjective comments that the residency program ensures lasting success.

References

1. DePasse JM, Palumbo MA, Eberson CP, Daniels AH. Academic characteristics of orthopaedic surgery residency applicants from 2007 to 2014. J Bone Joint Surg Am. 2016;98(9):788–95.
2. Raman T, Alrabaa RG, Sood A, Maloof P, Benevenia J, Berberian W. Does residency selection criteria predict performance in orthopaedic surgery residency? Clin Orthop Relat Res. 2016;474(4):908–14.
3. Turner NS, Shaughnessy WJ, Berg EJ, Larson DR, Hanssen AD. A quantitative composite scoring tool for orthopaedic residency screening and selection. Clin Orthop Relat Res. 2006;449:50–5.
4. Black KP, Abzug JM, Chinchilli VM. Orthopaedic in-training examination scores: a correlation with USMLE results. J Bone Joint Surg Am. 2006;88(3):671–6.
5. Dougherty PJ, Walter N, Schilling P, Najibi S, Herkowitz H. Do scores of the USMLE Step 1 and OITE correlate with the ABOS Part I certifying examination?: a multicenter study. Clin Orthop Relat Res. 2010;468(10):2797–802.

  6. Dirschl DR, Dahners LE, Adams GL, Crouch JH, Wilson FC. Correlating selection criteria with subsequent performance as residents. Clin Orthop Relat Res. 2002;399:265–71.
  7. Evarts CM. Resident selection: a key to the future of orthopaedics. Clin Orthop Relat Res. 2006;449:39–43.
  8. Bandiera G, Regehr G. Reliability of a structured interview scoring instrument for a Canadian postgraduate emergency medicine training program. Acad Emerg Med. 2004;11(1):27–32.
  9. ACGME program requirements for graduate medical education in orthopaedic surgery [Internet]. 2016 [updated 2015 Sept 27; cited 2016 Aug 31] https://www.acgme.org/Portals/0/PFAssets/ ProgramRequirements/260_orthopaedic_surgery_2016.pdf.
 10. Gil JA, Daniels AH, Weiss AP. Variability in surgical case volume of orthopaedic surgery residents: 2007 to 2013. J Am Acad Orthop Surg. 2016;24(3):207–12.
 11. Hinds RM, Gottschalk MB, Capo JT. National trends in carpal tunnel release and hand fracture procedures performed during orthopaedic residency: an analysis of ACGME case logs. J Grad Med Educ. 2016;8(1):63–7.
 12. Gil JA, Waryasz GR, Owens BD, Daniels AH. Variability of arthroscopy case volume in orthopaedic surgery residency. Arthroscopy. 2016;32(5):892–7.
 13. Orthopaedic surgery minimum numbers. http://www.acgme.org/ portals/0/pfassets/programresources/260_ors_case_log_minimum_numbers.pdf.
 14. Jeray KJ, Frick SL. A survey of resident perspectives on surgical case minimums and the impact on milestones, graduation, credentialing, and preparation for practice: AOA critical issues. J Bone Joint Surg Am. 2014;96(23):e195.
 15. Gil JA, Daniels AH, Akelman E. Resident exposure to peripheral nerve surgical procedures during residency training. J Grad Med Educ. 2016;8(2):173–9.
 16. VanHeest A, Kuzel B, Agel J, Putnam M, Kalliainen L, Fletcher J. Objective structured assessment of technical skill in upper extremity surgery. J Hand Surg Am. 2012;37(2):332–7. 7 e1–4
 17. Anderson DD, Long S, Thomas GW, Putnam MD, Bechtold JE, Karam MD. Objective Structured Assessments of Technical Skills (OSATS) does not assess the quality of the surgical result effectively. Clin Orthop Relat Res. 2016;474(4):874–81.
 18. Wongworawat MD. Editor's Spotlight/Take 5: Objective Structured Assessments of Technical Skills (OSATS) does not

assess the quality of the surgical result effectively. Clin Orthop Relat Res. 2016;474(4):871–3.

19. Clement RC, Olsson E, Katti P, Esther RJ. Fringe benefits among US Orthopedic residency programs vary considerably: a national survey. HSS J. 2016;12(2):158–64.

20. Anderson RW. The need for research training in orthopaedic residency education. Clin Orthop Relat Res. 2006;449:81–8.

21. Konstantakos EK, Laughlin RT, Markert RJ, Crosby LA. Assuring the research competence of orthopedic graduates. J Surg Educ. 2010;67(3):129–34.

22. Stern PJ, Albanese S, Bostrom M, Day CS, Frick SL, Hopkinson W, et al. Orthopaedic surgery milestones. J Grad Med Educ. 2013;5(1 Suppl 1):36–58.

23. Bradley KE, Andolsek KM. A pilot study of orthopaedic resident self-assessment using a milestones' survey just prior to milestones implementation. Int J Med Educ. 2016;7:11–8.

24. Ibrahim H, Stadler DJ, Archuleta S, Shah NG, Bertram A, Nair SC, et al. Clinician-educators in emerging graduate medical education systems: description, roles and perceptions. Postgrad Med J. 2016;92(1083):14–20.

25. Grant RE, Murphy LA, Murphy JE. Expansion of the coordinator role in orthopaedic residency program management. Clin Orthop Relat Res. 2008;466(3):737–42.

26. Roberts SM, Jarvis-Selinger S, Pratt DD, Polonijo A, Stacy E, Wisener K, et al. Reshaping orthopaedic resident education in systems-based practice. J Bone Joint Surg Am. 2012;94(15):e1131–7.

27. Alman BA, Ferguson P, Kraemer W, Nousiainen MT, Reznick RK. Competency-based education: a new model for teaching orthopaedics. Instr Course Lect. 2013;62:565–9.

28. Swanson D, Marsh JL, Hurwitz S, DeRosa GP, Holtzman K, Bucak SD, et al. Utility of AAOS OITE scores in predicting ABOS part I outcomes: AAOS exhibit selection. J Bone Joint Surg Am. 2013;95(12):e84.

29. Ponce B, Savage J, Momaya A, Seales J, Oliver J, McGwin G, et al. Association between orthopaedic in-training examination subsection scores and ABOS Part I examination performance. South Med J. 2014;107(12):746–50.

30. Thordarson DB, Ebramzadeh E, Sangiorgio SN, Schnall SB, Patzakis MJ. Resident selection: how we are doing and why? Clin Orthop Relat Res. 2007;459:255–9.

31. Overview of Board Certification [Internet]. [cited 2016 Aug 31]. https://www.abos.org/certification/board-certification.aspx.

32. ACGME Resident Survey—Program FAQs [Internet]. 2015 [updated 2015; cited 2016 Aug 31]. http://www.acgme.org/Portals/0/ACGME_Resident_Survey-Program_FAQs.pdf.
33. ACGME Resident Survey Content Areas [Internet]. 2014 [updated 2014; cited 2016 Aug 31]. http://www.acgme.org/Portals/0/ResidentSurvey_ContentAreas.pdf.
34. ACGME Faculty Survey—Program FAQs [Internet]. 2015 [updated 2015; cited 2016 Aug 31]. http://www.acgme.org/Portals/0/ACGME_Faculty_Survey-Program_FAQs.pdf.
35. ACGME Faculty Survey Question Content Areas [Internet]. 2015 [updated 2015; cited 2016 Aug 31]. http://www.acgme.org/Portals/0/ACGME%20FacultySurvey%20QuestionContentAreas.pdf.
36. Case Log Guidelines: Review Committee for Orthopaedic Surgery [Internet]. 2014 [updated 2014; cited 2016 Aug 31] http://www.acgme.org/portals/0/pfassets/programresources/260_case_log_guidelines.pdf.
37. Dwyer T, Glover Takahashi S, Kennedy Hynes M, Herold J, Wasserstein D, Nousiainen M, et al. How to assess communication, professionalism, collaboration and the other intrinsic CanMEDS roles in orthopedic residents: use of an objective structured clinical examination (OSCE). Can J Surg. 2014;57(4):230–6.
38. Phillips D, Zuckerman JD, Strauss EJ, Egol KA. Objective structured clinical examinations: a guide to development and implementation in orthopaedic residency. J Am Acad Orthop Surg. 2013;21(10):592–600.
39. Bernard JA, Dattilo JR, Srikumaran U, Zikria BA, Jain A, LaPorte DM. Reliability and validity of 3 methods of assessing orthopedic resident skill in shoulder surgery. J Surg Educ. 2016;
40. Zuckerman JD, Holder JP, Mercuri JJ, Phillips DP, Egol KA. Teaching professionalism in orthopaedic surgery residency programs. J Bone Joint Surg Am. 2012;94(8):e51.
41. DeRosa GP. Professionalism and virtues. Clin Orthop Relat Res. 2006;449:28–33.
42. Kim JJ, Gifford ED, Moazzez A, Sidwell RA, Reeves ME, Hartranft TH, et al. Program factors that influence American Board of Surgery in-Training Examination Performance: a multi-institutional study. J Surg Educ. 2015;72(6):e236–42.
43. Jacobs JS, Roberta E. Journey to authenticity: voices of chief residents. Chicago: ARC; 2007.

Chapter 12
Conclusion

Barbara L. Joyce and Paul J. Dougherty

We hope this book has provided a wide range of practical ideas that can be implemented in your program, and stimulated your thinking about orthopaedic surgery education. Orthopaedic surgery training has been experiencing a transformational shift from an apprenticeship model of education to a competency-based model of education. *The Orthopaedic Educator: A Pocket Guide* was designed to provide orthopaedic surgery faculty and program directors with an easy-to-use, practical, and concise guide focused on orthopaedic surgery education that would help program directors and faculty navigate this change. Chapters on curricular design and methods of assessment highlighted frameworks that can be used to design outcome-based training programs. Innovative ideas, such as the chapter on a Musculoskeletal Medicine

B.L. Joyce, PhD (✉)
Oakland University William Beaumont School of Medicine,
446 O'Dowd Hall, 2200 N. Squirrel Road,
Rochester, MI 48307, USA
e-mail: joyce@oakland.edu

P.J. Dougherty, MD
Department of Orthopaedic Surgery,
University of Florida College of Medicine—Jacksonville,
655 W 8th Street, 2nd Floor ACC, Jacksonville, FL 32209, USA
e-mail: paul.dougherty@jax.ufl.edu

© Springer International Publishing AG 2018
P.J. Dougherty, B.L. Joyce (eds.), *The Orthopedic Educator*,
DOI 10.1007/978-3-319-62944-5_12

Clerkship, highlight the evolution of third-year training of medical students.

While the landscape of orthopaedic educational training is rapidly changing, many constants remain. The importance of teaching operative and nonoperative skills and providing targeted feedback for resident improvement has always been at the forefront of training. The practical strategies provided here offered a framework for teaching and providing feedback and can be customized to an individual program. The chapter on remediating residents provided an overall framework for determining a stepwise process and structure for remediation of a resident within a residency program. Strategies and examples for designing successful faculty development programs that address the needs of orthopaedic educators have been presented. Because of the increasing complexity of residency, faculty development programs will become more important to provide faculty with the knowledge and skills to create strong educational programs.

Unfortunately, a "one-size-fits-all" approach will not work for programs. Programs are unique microsystems, and each program will have to select the best curricula, assessment tools, faculty development strategies, etc. for their particular program. Hopefully, readers have found throughout the chapters contained in the book some practical ideas to address their educational programming needs. Much work still needs to be done to develop reliable and valid assessment tools, best practices for faculty development, and best practices for teaching surgical skills. As the field moves forward, educators and scholars will need to effectively collaborate and disseminate their work to benefit the greater medical educational community.

Index

© Springer International Publishing AG 2018
P.J. Dougherty, B.L. Joyce (eds.), *The Orthopedic Educator*,
DOI 10.1007/978-3-319-62944-5

Made in the USA
Monee, IL
07 July 2026